PREGNANCY PAIN

Fix Your Pain and Become the Boss of Your Body
Tips and Tricks from a Physical Therapist and Mother

DR. LAURA SANNER

ISBN Paperback: 978-1-7356061-0-1
ISBN E-book: 978-1-7356061-1-8

HEALTH ADVICE DISCLAIMER

This book intends to provide helpful general information on the subjects that it addresses. Examples of injuries and their prognosis are based on typical representations of those injuries. The information given is not intended as representations of every individual's potential injury.

It is not in any way a substitute for the advice of the reader's own physicians or other medical professionals based on the reader's own individual conditions, symptoms, or concerns. As with any medical issue, each person's symptoms can vary. Each person's recovery from injury can also vary, depending upon background, previous medical history, application of exercises, motivation to follow advice, and various other physical factors.

It is impossible to give a completely accurate diagnosis and prognosis without a thorough physical examination, and likewise the advice given for management of an injury cannot be deemed fully accurate in the absence of this examination. No guarantees of specific results are expressly made or implied in this book.

This book is intended for general education purposes only. It does not serve as medical advice or a treatment plan. Do not use this book to replace going to your own healthcare professional. Consult with your doctors or healthcare professionals before doing the activities outlined in this book. By reading this book, you agree to hold harmless and indemnify the author and publisher for any and all injuries resulting from any and all claims that arise from your use or misuse of the directions or suggestions given in this book.

The author is a certified physical therapist and not a medical doctor. The content in this publication is provided for informational purposes and is not intended as medical advice or recommending specific treatment to individuals. Consult your health providers if you are experiencing any symptoms or if you have any health concerns. This information is not a substitute for professional medical advice, diagnosis or treatment. By using any and all of this information you do so at your own risk. No warranties are expressed or implied by the information contained in this publication. Any application of the material provided is at the reader's discretion and is their sole responsibility.

DEDICATION

This book is dedicated to:

My husband T.J.: My cheerleader and rock, day in and day out.

My parents and brother, Andy: The first cheerleaders I ever had.

My daughters: They make me the mom and woman I am today.

My family, friends and patients: For kicking my butt and asking me the hard questions, so I can deliver the best answers.

I love you all.

FREE CHEAT SHEET!

Moms deserve gifts! As a thank you for purchasing my book, I'm providing you with a free Cheat Sheet.

It covers the key ideas from this book. Visit www.pregnancypainbook.com/cheatsheet for printable exercise pictures, and step by step instructions and tips from desk posture to kinesio taping so you have a quick, easy to use guide.

CONTENTS

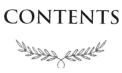

INTRODUCTION

You are having a baby! Or you're getting your body ready to have a baby!

Maybe your body hurts, or perhaps you don't want your body to start hurting. Either way, this is the book for you.

This is your fast pass to prevent or minimize your back and joint pain. By incorporating these techniques into your life, you'll solve common pregnancy problems. I'll show you how to support your body, stretch it when it's tight, and make it stronger to reduce and prevent pain.

This is not the book for you if you're a mother of five that has pregnancy pain handled. You don't need these tips.

Why should you read this book? Because if you wait, you could have pain that overshadows your joy. Don't be the pregnant lady that can't move. Be the pregnant lady that wows your friends. Be the mom that takes action and does it right away.

As a mother of two, I've had pain with pregnancy. As a Physical Therapist, I used what I knew to help myself. I managed the pain I had in my lower back, all while continuing to work—and chasing a toddler! Since then, I've answered hundreds of questions about exercises, posture, natural healing, and where/when to spend your money on the must-have gear.

This book is your useful, accessible, "What would my PT say" guide that gets right to the good stuff in a direct and easy to follow manner.

I've tested everything to see what works and what doesn't. I've shared these tips with friends and patients, but it's all been in my head until now. In this book, I'll be able to share my expertise with you. I'll answer all the questions you have about pregnancy. And I won't let you waste your time on the epic fails I've had, like registering for a diaper bag for a husband who would never, in a million years, use one.

After reading my book, you'll have an easy-to-find list of these tips too. You'll have a plan of attack for your bad days and your good days. All pregnancies are filled with both.

My cousin Sarah was in her second trimester of pregnancy while I was writing this book. One day she mentioned that simple tasks like taking the dogs for a walk were plagued with annoyances. A mundane task like sneezing now caused a tinkle, which was never an issue before. Her husband affectionately called this "taking a trip to Tinkle Town." Sarah just wanted it to stop. By adding some of these exercises to her routine, she reduced her trips to Tinkle Town. A win, for sure!

After you read this book, you will better understand how your body moves. Even more importantly, you'll have a plan to move and feel better. The exercises, posture, and gear you're about to master are proven to create positive, lasting results.

You're the boss of your body. Learn more about what's going on inside of it right now. Take control and put the discomfort behind you. Experience the joy you are meant to have.

CHAPTER ONE

MOVE WITH LESS PAIN

POSTURE, SLEEP SET UP, AND EASY FIXES TO START TODAY

Five rounded blades of the off-white ceiling fan go round and round. Salty summer air swirls through the room. The gentle breeze from the fan brushes my fly-aways from my ponytail across my cheek. My toes stretch to the very bottom of the sheet, and my back makes a deep 'thunk'.

I was ten weeks pregnant with my second child and my back was *stiff*. This didn't happen with the first. Why was my body hurting like this, ten weeks into my second?

I've felt like a broken record sharing my stories with friends and patients. I've solved your problem before. Let's make your pregnancy journey active and less painful. Let's get started!

POSTURE

Posture is the number one topic that makes me feel like a broken record.

I hear, "I know I have bad posture, but what should I do to fix it?"

And I reply, over and over, "Which posture or activity hurts you the most? Point to where it hurts."

Answer that question for yourself. Is it sleep, getting in and out of bed or a car, working on your computer or phone, driving or sitting for a long time? And what does that activity hurt? Which specific muscle or joint? Point to where it hurts.

Posture is the position of the body. When you're pregnant, your weight, center of gravity, and posture change, which means "good posture" for every activity is going to change, too. By being aware of these changes, you can help alleviate unnecessary pain.

In this section, I'll cover the areas where you can make little changes to get the most out of your efforts. The cool thing is that once these little changes become your new normal, you don't have to think about it anymore. It's not a chore to have good posture. Your new normal just feels better.

I've outlined below how to approach sleeping, getting in and out of bed, and romance so they hurt less for you. I separated these from sitting and walking activities; continue on to the next chapter for those tips.

SLEEP

The top sleep position for pregnant women—and, furthermore, people in general—is on your side.[1] The ideal line up for sleeping posture is keeping your spine in a straight line. How to keep your spine straight varies from person to person, and you often need support to achieve this.

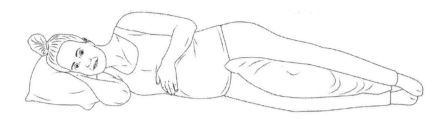

Sleeping on your side

The Best Sleep Posture

Try This: Lie on your side. Get comfortable. Where is your top leg? Is it staying perfectly on top of your bottom leg? Do you roll your top leg forward? Typically, rolling the top leg forward happens as you relax your muscles and let gravity win. Think about your spine now. Is it in a straight line?

Your lower back probably twisted to allow your hip to fall forward. As you twist, you compress the bottom of your spine, and open up the top. Doing so takes your spine out of alignment, and can cause pain (or adds to it), especially if you hold that position for a long time while sleeping.

Now try this: Take a spare pillow and put that between your knees. Is it as easy for the top leg to fall forward? It shouldn't be. Putting a pillow between your knees helps keep the lower back in a straight, or neutral position. It can also soften the pressure from one knee to the other, if you're worried about knee pain.

If you're petite like me, you can use a big, fluffy comforter instead of a pillow. Personally, I found that a pillow was too bulky and jacked up my top hip too high. If adding a body pillow to the mix makes you hurt worse, it's probably too fluffy and round for you.

The comforter fit best for me, but there is also a special Knee Pillow for Side Sleepers that has solved the 'wake up with pain' problem for many of my patients. It provides the stability and support of pregnancy pillows without pushing your partner out of bed.

The uber-supporting pregnancy pillows are often massive. The knee pillow also travels well. Be careful though. Your partner might steal it!

Still not sure if you're doing it right? Take a picture of your set-up from above. If you trace the outline of your entire spine, is it in a straight line? If you're having pain when you wake up and the line isn't quite straight, keep making improvements for yourself.

Does sleeping on your side cause you shoulder pain?
A body pillow may be the answer. Or, alternatively, one pillow between your legs and another pillow to hug. Keep in mind that separate pillows are more likely to end up on the floor, though. Resting your top arm on a pillow keeps your shoulder in line with your body, instead of letting it fall too far forward.

Need a break from side sleeping—maybe to get a little pressure off of the outside of your hips in the earlier months of pregnancy? The next-best choice is lying on your back. Keep the same principles in mind: you want a straight spine. This is an option up until week 20, then side lying is how you should spend your nights.[2]

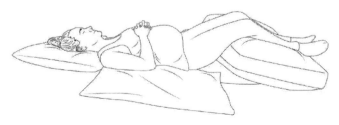

Sleeping on your back

Try a pillow or small bolster under your knees, and a towel roll or pillow under your arms for extra support. Lying on your back lets your shoulders fall too far behind their natural position otherwise.

In the third trimester, avoid laying on your back longer than five minutes. The inferior vena cava is the vein that gets smooshed by your uterus in this position, restricting oxygen to the baby and putting undue strain on your kidneys. With adjustable beds, you should still avoid sleeping on your back even if your head and/or legs are elevated, as gravity still presses the baby straight down.

Do your hands fall asleep when you sleep? They could feel tingly like pins and needles, numb like you are wearing a glove that's too tight, or heavy and slow moving. If your shoulders hurt or your arms or fingers tingle, try a small pillow under your upper arm bone (humerus) to lift your arm and bring it in line with the midline of your rib cage.

For me, this wasn't a major problem until pregnancy. The likely reason is that your body gets swollen during pregnancy due to an increased pressure on the nerves and veins in the front of your shoulders. These nerves run all the way down to your fingers. It could also be caused by increased pressure in your wrists.

If it comes on gradually, it's usually nothing to worry about. If it comes on suddenly and the numbness doesn't go away as your day gets going, mention it to your doctor. You can wear a splint on your hand to keep your wrists from moving too much to take the pressure off your hands if the tingling is driving you crazy.

If limiting movement doesn't appeal to you or it makes it worse, try this:

1. Gently squeeze your hands into fists ten times.
2. Slowly bend your elbows then straighten them, ten times.
3. Roll your shoulders forward, slowly, ten times.
4. Roll your shoulders backward, slowly, ten times.
5. Roll to a new position.
6. Whichever part of the list helped most, do that part again as many times as you want.

Sleep Position to Avoid

What's the worst sleeping position when pregnant (or in general)? On your stomach! This takes up all the extra space between the bones in your back, and the compression through the night can strain everything from your legs, back, neck, to even your jaw.

When you lie down to go to bed, start on your side or back. If you wake up and find you're on your stomach, or in a position that hurts, move! Fix it. Go back to sleep. Repeat.

New habits take repetition to stick. I find improving your sleep posture is a habit that takes longer to correct, since you can't consciously fix a bad set up when you're asleep and unconscious. Stick with it, and eventually your body will learn.

Fix it. Go back to sleep.

How Many Pillows Should I Have Under My Head?

The short answer: however many you need to keep your spine in a straight line. My ideal set-up is one when I'm on my back and two thin pillows when I'm on my side, but yours may be completely different.

Indeed, even my own set-up changed completely when I changed my bed. When our memory-foam bed got worn out, the bed we replaced it with was so much more firm. I used the same pillows, and after a few nights, I woke up with a kink in my neck so fierce I couldn't turn my head to the left at all.

The solution? I got a new pillow! Turns out this core pillow is perfect for people like me that alternate from side to back to side. It has a divot cut out in the middle for your head to rest in when you're on your back, and high sides to support your head when you're on your side. It took a few sleeps to get used to, but it works great if you have a firmer bed.

Do you wake up with pain? Do you feel the stiffest in the morning?

First, try to use one of those tips I just outlined for the best set-up.

Second, there are some exercises to do before you get out of bed (if you need a bathroom break, take that first, then slide back into bed!). See Chapter 5 for Bed Stretches.

GETTING OUT OF (AND INTO) BED

As your pregnancy progresses, you're likely to notice that even simple tasks, such as climbing out of bed, can be difficult. This can be further complicated by your more frequent trips to the bathroom each night as your uterus encroaches on your bladder. By following these steps, you're likely to save yourself unnecessary pain.

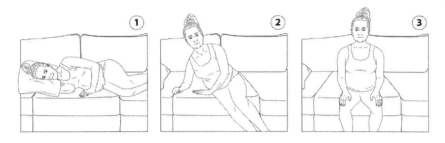

Log Roll

The "Log Roll": Five Basic Steps for Getting Out of Bed
- Tighten your abdominal muscles first.
- Roll onto your side, with bent knees.
- Push upright with your arms.
- Swing your feet to the floor. Wait to make sure you're not dizzy.
- Stand up.

ROMANCE

It's important to note that you can be intimate with your significant other for the entire length of your pregnancy. It is not going to hurt the baby if you keep the following things in mind. The further you get into your nine months, the more creative you may have to get with positions.

The most important rule of thumb is, as with all forms of exercise, if it causes high pain levels, stop doing it that way. If it works for you, do more of that!

Positions to Avoid

Avoid being on the bottom after the 20th week, as this can compress the blood flow to you and the baby. As with sleep posture, laying on your stomach for intimacy can also be uncomfortable and press on your belly.

Avoid lying on your stomach from about the third month of pregnancy to delivery. Your growing baby is no longer protected by your pelvis.

Particularly in the last trimester and for the first two months postpartum, skip being on all fours. If your butt is elevated above your head, your uterus can move up toward your head. When that happens, air can enter your blood stream through the open placental site.

This is called air embolism. This air bubble in your vein is rare, but dangerous. These air bubbles can travel to other areas of your body and may cause respiratory failure, a stroke, or heart attack.[3]

If you've had bleeding or other symptoms of placenta detachment occur during pregnancy, all-fours is a hard "no". For the same reasons, never blow air into your vagina while you're pregnant or for the eight weeks following childbirth, as this can also cause an air embolism.

Bleeding after sex can happen, especially in the first trimester. It could be a sign of natural changes to your cervix, but definitely tell your doc. They may recommend taking a break for a few weeks until that stops happening.

Getting uterus contractions or cramps during or after intimacy is also probably nothing to worry about, but in rare cases it could be more serious. Share any new pains you're having with your OB.

Chapter 1 Key Points
- Side sleeping is best.
- Log roll every single time you get into and out of bed.
- If you hurt, move or fix it.
- Romance is OK through the third trimester if you make a few adjustments.

CHAPTER TWO

SITTING AND WALKING WITH LESS PAIN

One third of your life is spent in bed, and another third is spent on your feet! Read on if you're desperate to find the best shoes to wear for the next nine months. I'll also cover little changes that really add up to less pain in your day.

SHOES

Your body is a tower. Your feet are the base of your tower. If the base is unstable, everything above will have more stress and strain. Wear supportive shoes to provide a stable base for all the joints above your feet.

Do you own flip-flops in every color of the rainbow? Me too! At least, Old Laura did. Old Laura also had back pain after standing or shopping for as little as three hours.

Flip flops became popular summer shoes in the 1950s and 60s due to their convenience. They're great for the pool or when you have sand between your toes, but the average American logs about 5,000 steps per day (20,000 with an active job), so we need a little more support than cheap, colorful beach shoes can offer.[4]

I've since thrown out all but a couple pairs of flip flops. New Laura just wears flip flops to the pool or beach, and New Laura's back feels *much* better.

Feet hit the ground and then push off with each step in three different ways. If you look at the soles of your shoes, you might find evidence of wear that helps you identify which of these categories you fall into.

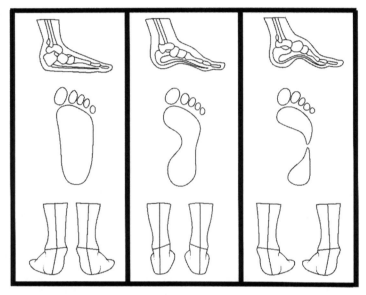

Types of Feet: A) Overpronator, B) Neutral, C) Supinator

Overpronator: If you can see a tilt inward or more wear toward the inside curve of your shoe, you may be an overpronator. This foot rolls too far inward when bearing the weight of your body. You're likely suited for a motion control shoe.

Neutral: With a neutral foot, you land on the outer edge of the foot, roll inward, then push off on the outside of your foot again. The wear and tear on your shoes is more even from the inside to outside edges. You are looking for a neutral shoe.

Supinator AKA Under-Pronator: You tend to have high arches and walk or run on the outer edges of your feet. As such, the outer edges of your shoes likely show the most wear and tear. A cushioning shoe is your best fit.

A physical therapist can help you find the types of shoe that are best for you. Alternately, if you have a local shoe store that specializes in sensible shoes, running shoes, or otherwise putting you in the right shoe, I always recommend a visit.

You'll pay a couple extra bucks for their experience, but it's worth it. The good stores often have a two-week return period. I did actually cash in on their return period once; the second pair they selected for me was *it!* I've stayed in that brand and style of shoe for years and years since. After you discover your perfect shoe match, online shopping becomes an option when it's time for your next pair.

Other Pro Tips:

Don't make a pair of shoes multitask. Your work shoes should not be your work-out shoes. The material that makes up the sole gets squished during the day and needs time to recover between uses. After a 30 minute workout, a shoe is 40% deformed, and takes 24 hours to recover.

If you wear high heels, a 2¼-inch limit is recommended by the American Podiatric Medical Association.

Make sure you have enough room to wiggle your toes. Each brand has a different "average foot shape" model. If your foot is wide across the toes, you'll like shoes with a bigger toe box like New Balance. If you have a narrow foot, you might prefer Nike. If you're like me, Brooks is the best fit. Funny enough, separate from my shoe journey, my brother also swears by Brooks. You can't outrun your genetics!

Research varies, but 300-500 miles is the running shoe industry standard for when shoes lose their cushioning and support. There are variables like the runner's weight or the terrain where you're running that can affect the wear and tear of shoes. The industry also says to replace your shoes every six to eight months, but again, that can vary.[5]

The tread may still look pretty good, but the foam can wear out faster. If your "dogs are barking" (AKA feet hurt), or a different body part hurts more than usual, it's likely time for a new pair.

SITTING

Since so many of us spend a good chunk of time sitting, it's important to consider your position. In fact, besides sleeping, computer set-up is the most common posture question I get.

Maybe you're putting in longer hours now to bank time or money so you can enjoy a longer maternity leave. Your muscles are tired. There's never been a better time to listen to your body and do a thorough posture check.

Computer Posture

Here is the best way to fit your workstation around you. You may need to readjust as your belly grows in the next nine months, but these tips will be relevant for you today, and forever.

- o Take breaks! Set a timer to stand up, stretch, or walk a lap around your desk or hallway every 20 minutes.
- o If you're unable to get up due to a meeting or work task, at minimum move your hips as if doing a seated hula hoop. Then

roll your shoulders back, turn your head side to side, point your toes up and down, march your legs, and resettle using the tips below.

o Settle your shoulder blades. The back of your shoulders should rest on the back of your chair. Avoid an arched back or hunched shoulders. Find a chair with a backrest, not just a stool.

o Bring the ground to you. Adjust your seat height so that your knees are slightly below your hips with your feet resting comfortably on the floor. An angle slightly greater than 90° for your knees is best. Often, this will require adjusting the height of the seat. This might even mean putting something under your feet: a footstool, phone book, or empty box.

- I actually duct-taped two phone books together and wrote LAURA on them in super-big letters. It kept footrest poachers away for sure. My personal footrest is still in use under my desk at work. I made it years ago. Now that phone books are all but nonexistent, you could do the same thing with some old books, or a sturdy shoe box.

o Sit up straight. Not overly straight, but like a string is attached to the tippy top of your head and you're being gently pulled up. Now scoot back and check how the chair fits to your body. If there are gaps, or you have to tighten your muscles or sag your body to fit into the chair, the backrest needs some help. Use a lumbar roll or roll up a hand towel and place this at the small of your back. Test out different thicknesses of the roll and change its height until you feel your back muscles can relax.

- Most adjustable rolling chairs will have a backrest. It should support your back from your mid-pelvis to mid-shoulder blade.

- You'll need to adjust this as your belly grows and pulls your spine into a more arched angle.

o Rest your arms. Make sure your forearms are parallel to the floor and your elbows are at about a 90° angle. Your forearms should rest on chair arms or on your desk to take up the weight of your upper body. If you skip this step, the tension will creep into your upper trapezius muscles, where your head connects to your shoulders. It only takes one hour of missing arm support for knots to form in these muscles!

o Adjust so your eyes are looking forward. Prop documents up using a document holder stand between the keyboard and your monitor if you have a lot to copy from paper to computer.

o Adopt correct mouse and keyboard positioning. Keep your mouse near the keyboard so you don't have to reach far for it. Reaching for the mouse can over-stretch and tire out your muscles. If you're having a lot of wrist pain, my patients that switch to a vertical mouse love them.

  - The keyboard height should be at or just below your elbow height. The front portion of the keyboard can be raised slightly to prevent your wrists from bending.
  - Keep your wrists straight, not bent up, down, or crooked to the side, with your elbows at your sides. A split or wave-style keyboard is a nice splurge.

If you are fighting with wrist, neck or shoulder pain, consider some of those ergonomic upgrades. Your changing body might have brought about these changes, but the upgrades will make your life better for years to come.

Watch for problems. Pay attention to warning signs like headaches, fatigue, muscle pain, or cramping. If you get any of these, keep testing one change at a time.

Use the Computer Posture tips above for anything you do sitting down. This includes texting, meetings, writing, studying, or even watching TV.

Text Neck is a real thing. It's neck pain due to looking down for prolonged periods of time. Share these tips with your partner, friends, and future grandparents, too! They've got a lot of looking down to do with all the cute pictures you'll soon be sending.

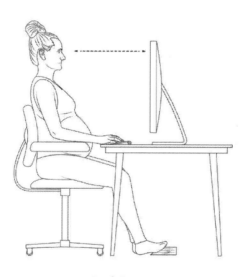

Desk Posture

DRIVING

Adjust the height of your rearview mirror and/or the distance of your seat to the foot pedals every 20 minutes for longer, painful commutes. This will reduce prolonged strain to your spine and body by gently changing up the angles of your joints.

When possible, you want to have equal weight through your legs. One thing that gave me sharp pain in my lower back was getting into and out of my car.

For pregnancy #1, I was driving a very low-to-the-ground 2002 Saturn. I called her Susie. By the middle of pregnancy #2, my husband and I put on our big girl and big boy pants and agreed it was time for the Mini Van life.

Getting into the van was harder for me, but getting out from a taller angle was easier. (By the way, my van still doesn't have a good name, though I've considered Millie.) Every car has its ups and downs.

Whether you're riding in a sporty, little car or a big, loud truck, follow these suggestions to avoid hurting yourself. I can attest that these techniques work for most vehicles.

Getting INTO a car
- o   Sit first.
- o   Keep your knees together.
- o   Pivot both legs into the car together.

Getting OUT of a car
- o   Keep your knees together.
- o   Pivot both legs out of the car.
- o   With both feet on the ground, stand up.

If you are still having pain standing all the way up tall, take some time to let your joints adjust from the sitting to standing position, especially if it was a longer or somewhat stressful drive. Shift your weight from side to side either while you're still in the car, or after you stand up.

Move your hips around as if you were hula-hooping to get your body moving and progress to your upright posture slowly.

This sounds like extra steps, but you have to move with care to avoid repeated strains. Try these steps every day, and note whether you start to hurt less.

Also, don't forget: you can use many of the tips from sitting at your desk when you're sitting in a vehicle. Take some time to move your legs and roll your shoulders to avoid getting stiff.

How to Wear Your Seatbelt

First, always wear your seatbelt so you and your baby are safer in the event of a car accident.[6]

Keep the car seat as upright as possible, not reclined. The lap belt should be low and flat on the top of your thighs, *under* your tummy. The shoulder belt should sit between your breasts.

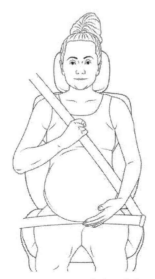

How to wear your seat belt while pregnant

In the event that you're in a crash, no matter how minor, get checked out. Call your doctor or visit the Emergency Room, even if you feel fine.

Chapter 2 Key Points
- It's OK to wear cute heels and flip flops, sometimes. Most of the time, wear good, supportive shoes.
- Bring the support to you when you're sitting.
- If you hurt, move or fix it.
- Take breaks every 20 minutes.

CHAPTER THREE

MEDICAL CONDITIONS

When I mentally committed to writing this book, I began interviewing everybody—moms, dads, future parents, grandparents, you name it. I asked them about their questions and the experiences they had.

My timing was impeccable. When I happened to be in for my annual check-in, I even got to interview my favorite OB-GYN, Dr. P. I'll start with the most common aches and pains according to his list (which very much matched what I was planning to put down). The tips covered in this book will help you fix each of these common ailments listed below.

COMMON ACHES AND PAINS

The aches and pains that you have are normal, but fixable. Keep that in mind now and as your body changes more and more.

You can manage your muscle imbalances and your pain with the strengthening and flexibility exercises in this book. If you're not yet pregnant, you can do the same exercises to give your body the best chance to eliminate future pregnancy pain.

Lower Back Pain

This is the most common orthopedic complaint during pregnancy. Depending on the study, 25-90% of women experience this during at least part of their pregnancy. Pregnancy related lower back pain usually begins between weeks 20 and 28 of gestation, but it may begin earlier.[7]

Hip Pain

Hip pain is another common complaint. I had outer-hip pain that was pretty bad during my final two months. When you lie on your side, there's not a lot of cushion between the surface of your hip bone and the bed. You might feel a sharp pain that won't completely go away when you change position.

Plantar Fasciitis

Plantar fasciitis is a sharp pulling pain felt on the bottom of your foot and in your heel. The classic sign is that the pain happens when you first put your feet down to stand up, after you've been sitting or lying for a while. Many women struggle with this later in pregnancy due to the increased pressure on the ligaments in their feet.

Sciatica

The sciatic nerve is the largest nerve in the body. It travels from the lower back down the back of the leg into the foot. When the nerve is pinched, you have "sciatica". In other words, it is pain running down the back of the leg, caused by a problem in the back. Sciatica sufferers may experience pain, numbness, tingling, and/or heaviness in the leg.

Many that suffer from lower back pain also get sciatica. Some people can even get sciatica but skip the actual pain in their lower back.

Arm Pain

Pins and needles in the arms and hands rounds out the aches and pains list. Similar to pregnancy changing your joint angles in your back, the same can happen in your neck. The upper back is stretched, and the back of the neck is tight, and this puts pressure on the nerves in your hands. Your arms or hands could feel pain, numb, tingly or heavy from something going on in your neck.

Carpal Tunnel syndrome has a pretty high prevalence during pregnancy as well. You may feel it in one hand or, like roughly half of those with Carpal Tunnel syndrome, you'll experience this in both hands.[8] It comes on gradually and feels like off and on numbness or tingling on the thumb and index finger side of your hand.

To get an official diagnosis, you need an electrodiagnostic test. This is somewhat invasive and painful. Needle probes are placed in your skin along your arm to check how well different parts of the nerve are working.

Instead, if you notice your hands burning or hurting during sleep, computer time, or another activity, bounce back to Chapters 1 and 2 for help with your posture. Night splints for your wrists can have a lot of positive impact.

Carpal tunnel pins and needles is a nerve pain. Keep your nerves moving freely by flexing and extending your wrists ten times when these feelings arise. As always, a physical therapist is a great resource if the pain is persisting.

SPINAL CURVE

Spines have a normal curve, wherein the small of your back gently arches, your middle to upper back rounds forward, and at your neck it gently arches again. Your center of gravity is like an invisible string that keeps you sitting tall.

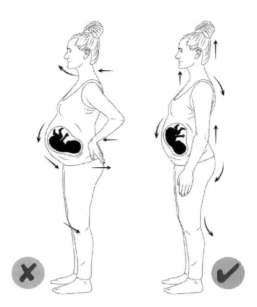

Spinal curves: a) Strained: Arched back, shoulders slumped forward. B) Better: An imaginary string helping you stand with your chest up and belly button in.

News Flash! Pregnancy changes your curves. The center of gravity shifts up and forward due to your uterus and breasts getting larger. Also, your hips rotate out a little more than normal. This contributes to the "waddling" walk you get when you're pregnant. To compensate, you must lean back and shift your weight back to keep balanced.

Relaxin is a hormone produced at higher levels during pregnancy, which relaxes ligaments in the pelvis in preparation for birth. How else would your pre-baby body make room for a seven-plus-pound baby and the associated pregnancy weight without breaking you in half?

The bad side of relaxin is that it can make your joints a little "loosey-goosey" and unstable, therefore easier to strain. Each of your spine curves become more exaggerated with each trimester. The deeper curves tighten your back muscles and stretch out the back of your legs.

The daily exercises in the next two chapters will help you keep your joints and muscles gently moving to balance all these changes.

ROUND LIGAMENT PAIN

Have you gotten any "shot-in-the-gut" sharp pains in the lower, front part of your belly? You typically start to feel these during the second trimester. It is most likely your round ligament snapping. It's very common, and it's considered a normal feeling during pregnancy.

The round ligament connects the front part of your womb to your groin, where your legs attach to your pelvis. As your belly grows, this ligament is overstretched and can easily be plucked with a change in position. These sharp, quickly resolving pains are normal.

What do you do? Keep your eyes peeled in Chapter 5. Try both the Seated Lower Back Stretch and the Double Knee to Chest Stretch. Of those two, pick your favorite. Do that exercise daily. Additionally, from that chapter, the abdominal bracing can reduce your ligament pain as well.

Also, s… l… o… w… d… o… w… n. If you usually blast through life and rush from one thing to the next, slow down. Take smaller steps, make smaller turns. Change positions slowly to put less tension on this ligament.

Warning sign: If any of these pains don't seem to be related to movement, time of day, or before or after meals, add it to the list of things you talk to your doctor about!

DIASTASIS RECTI

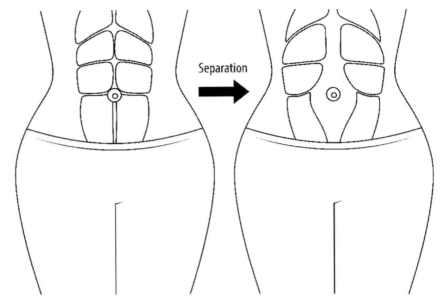

Separation

A) Normal abdominal muscle spacing, B) Diastasis recti separation

Diastasis recti separation, AKA ab separation, AKA split abs, AKA Mommy Belly, AKA Mummy Tummy, AKA Mommy Pooch, is another common pregnancy problem. The abdominal muscle closest to the surface of your belly is called rectus abdominis.

Really fit people can exercise these and get a "six pack." The major parts of this are the right and left recti muscles. These two halves join at the central seam, called the linea alba. When this seam pulls apart, like unzipping a zipper, you get an ab separation.

For some, it causes pain; for other's it does not. Many moms don't know about this condition (or that they have it). Some women who have a C-section have abdominal pain that they blame on their healing incisions.

Discomfort with your abs may be worse after eating or when you're trying to sleep. Getting out of bed or laying awkwardly with a sleeping infant may cause this pain to flare. Both my patients and my neighbors rave about how much better their backs, or abdominals felt after taking steps to address their diastasis recti, after they or their medical team identified the condition.

Think of the muscles in your body like a suit of armor. If your muscle has a gap in it, there is a chink in your armor. It weakens the whole suit and can be a factor in back pain now and in the future.

Why does this happen in pregnancy? Relaxin. That good and bad hormone again! The linea alba softens and the seam can split due to the pressure of the growing baby. There is also a genetic component to how soft or stretchy your tendons, ligaments and muscles are. Thus, some mamas are more prone to this split than others.

The separation can occur above, at, below the naval, or a combination of those areas. You may feel some discomfort in this area during the third trimester, but most women do not.

Of those who feel this separation, two thirds report it during the third trimester. Half as many report this during their six-week postpartum OB check.[9] This can also happen to men and non-pregnant women. It appears as a bulge when you bear down, like if you force something out when you're on the toilet.

How to check for it: Lie on your back with your knees bent. Do a crunch and lift your shoulders off the bed. Find the spot two inches above your navel. It is normal for this "zipper" to be about one centimeter wide, where you can place the width of one finger down the center of this line.

However, if you can fit the width of two fingers in the separation gap (two centimeters), that is positive or clinically significant. Welcome to the two-pack abs club.

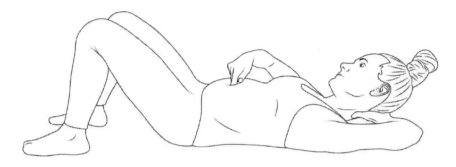

Diastasis recti self-check

Can I prevent or reduce this? Yes, prevention is key to management. Review the two Transverse Abdominal Exercises in Chapter 5 and discontinue your other "regular" ab workout to both prevent and to improve an existing separation. As a bonus, the better shape your ab muscles are in now, the more they can help push your baby out when it's go-time.

Exercising after the fact is not enough to bring the abs back together postpartum.[10] The good news is, you can help your abs heal after delivery by moving smarter. You can help the rectus muscles move toward the midline, and return closer to their intended position, instead of moving apart.

During everyday movements, lessen how hard you strain. All the tips from my first two chapters on posture keep working for you beyond pregnancy.

Doing your log-roll in and out of bed is one of the best things you can do for your abs on a daily basis. Remember, roll on to your side, then use your arm to help you push your body up to sitting.

Kinesiology tape can be a useful, temporary reminder and does help during pregnancy and after.[11] Use the Diastasis Recti taping in Chapter 10 for two to four weeks if you have a separation that is causing you abdominal or lower back discomfort. It will be your reminder while coaching yourself to move differently.

If you're sensitive to tape, and you're post-partum, an abdominal binder compression belt is a great alternative to help bring the muscles closer to where they should be.

ACID REFLUX

Most women, roughly 80%, have acid reflux, or GastroEsophageal Reflux Disease (GERD), during their pregnancy.[12] This especially shows up in heartburn. When stomach acid rises in the esophagus, the tube from your throat to your stomach, you might feel a burning sensation in your chest or lower throat.

Why?

Relaxin. Your favorite hormone! It not only relaxes your ligaments and muscles to make way for your growing baby, it also softens the muscles and valves that close off the esophagus from the stomach. Mix that with the newly cramped space in which your stomach lives, and you've got a recipe for acid back-flow.

A natural way to handle this is through lifestyle changes. In my early twenties, I had GERD. I even had an upper GI scope to check for damage. Luckily, all good. I'd tried daily prescription and over-the-counter pills. If I had a third big cup of coffee, the coffee won, and despite the medicine I'd have pretty bad heartburn that evening.

When I was trying to get pregnant, I tapered myself off the heartburn meds. And the coffee (which was the hardest thing for me to give up!). But even when I was pregnant and didn't drink coffee at all, I *still* had heartburn, and it was even worse. How unfair is that?

Some heartburn meds were listed as "probably safe" to use when pregnant. My cousin Sarah swears by Pepcid, which was recommended by her midwife, but I figured, why risk it if I could go "au naturel"?

I figured TUMS were ok, if I took them just "as needed". The problem was I got a little crazy with those, especially since they have the chewy ones now that taste like Starbursts. I'm the type that eats the yellow ones first to get them over with. Obviously pink are the best, I save those for last.

During one of my second trimester checkups, I told my OB I was taking maybe four to six TUMS a day. He said, "Whoa, whoa, whoa, stop the bus. The calcium in TUMS can give you kidney stones!" He reminded me of the goal I had abandoned: to calm my acid down with *no* medication.

Here's how I learned to manage my heartburn, meds-free:
- o Smaller meals and sips, more often.
- o Slow down: Eat slower to avoid overeating and overfilling your cramped stomach.
- o Avoid late-night snacks (if the baby will let you!). Finish eating two hours before you lie down. When you lie down, gravity cannot help keep your digestive juices in the stomach. Your stomach acid can more easily backflow up your esophagus.

o Keep a mental (or written, if you're a list-maker like me!) food journal. Everybody's food triggers are different. List the time of day, food eaten, and when and how bad the heartburn was. Seeing any trends?
  - Change up your foods. Is your acid worse after Taco Night? Your morning OJ + calcium?
  - Citrus, tomatoes, chocolate, fat, mint, and spicy foods are common triggers. See how you react to these foods especially, and adjust your diet accordingly.

Sleeping with Heartburn

Acid at night? Put blocks under the legs of your headboard to ramp up the top half of your bed. Risers under your bed legs work great. This will aid gravity in keeping those stomach juices where they belong and not travel up-hill so easily.

When elevating the head of your bed, higher is better, as long as you can still comfortably sleep on your side, with your spine in that nice straight line. Most people find that six to eight inches of elevation is the magic number.

Foods that Help

Apples and almonds became my go-to. Snacking on apples or high-fiber fruits and veggies 20 minutes before your main meal—or eating those first when you sit down to eat—can help work your acid in a good way so more of your food stays where it's supposed to after your meals.

You know what they say: "An apple a day…!" ~Welsh Proverb

HIGH RISK PREGNANCY

Being pregnant and having a baby goes as planned most of the time. Sometimes, however, you can hit some bumps in the road, which result in the pregnancy being considered high risk. The age you are while pregnant and previous medical issues are the main factors, but issues can also arise during a pregnancy, making it "high risk".

At 18 weeks, my first pregnancy was tagged as high risk. During the ultrasound when we found out if we were having a boy or a girl, the test found a white spot on the baby's heart. To monitor how her heart was working and developing, we had to go in for a *lot* of extra ultrasounds, at a place with a high-tech machine.

In the end, she was fine. But things like that may come up that the doctors want to keep an eye on.

As mentioned in the exercise and massage sections, those can be more aggressive treatment choices and should be avoided until you get the OK from your doc. The good news is that all the posture, gear, and other tips covered in this book are *always* super helpful, whether you are in the middle of a high-risk or smooth-sailing pregnancy.

Bed Rest

With certain conditions, your doctor may recommend bed rest later in your pregnancy.

"Bed rest" does not restrict *all* movements. If you lay without moving in bed for weeks, you will be really stiff!

When you're on bed rest for an orthopedic injury, I recommend modified bed rest. This means not lifting anything over ten pounds and avoiding any uncomfortable activity that lasts 20 minutes or more. Get up and stretch your legs hourly, at minimum.

You can and should move when on bed rest. The objective is to lessen the pressure on the umbilical cord, insertion, and uterus. Laying on your side, sitting, standing and shifting your weight, and being on hands and knees (as long as you don't put your chest on the ground) are OK in short bouts. Stick to 20 minutes or less for each at a time.

You can even do some exercise. However, if you feel nauseated or see any bleeding, those are red flags that you've overdone it.

Stay moving with activities that have a lower impact on your body. Run this outline by your doctor. Every pregnancy is different, and your doctor is your guide during this time.

And as always, listen to your body. If an activity makes you feel bad, stop.

Chapter 3 Key Points
- o   Review sleep posture from Chapter 1 if you're waking up with pain.
- o   Talk to your doc about sharp belly pains that are not related to activity.
- o   Slow down, take smaller steps, make smaller turns, and change positions slowly.
- o   Protect your ab muscles (for example, log roll in and out of bed).
- o   Think about and adjust what you're eating if you have acid reflux.
- o   If your pregnancy is high-risk, make a list of your specific movement/exercise questions for your doctor.

CHAPTER FOUR

Exercise You Can Start in Your First Trimester (or Before)

The Basics

There is a lot of conflicting information about exercising when pregnant. The problem is, if it could cause harm, no one wants to do a research study that would put a mom and/or their baby at risk. So the guidelines below are largely based on how our bodies work while doing these tasks and ways to make them safer during your pregnancy.

Exercise during pregnancy is OK. Read through these do's and don'ts to stay safe and healthy.

GENERAL PRE NATAL EXERCISE GUIDELINES

Fifteen to thirty minutes of mild to moderate exercise most days of the week is recommended when you're pregnant.

Disclaimer reminder: If you or the baby have any risk factors, double check with your doc.

From the American College of Obstetricians and Gynecologists (ACOG): "Generally, participation in a wide range of recreational activities appears to be safe during pregnancy; however, each sport should be reviewed individually for its potential risk, and activities with a high risk of abdominal trauma should be avoided during pregnancy. Scuba diving also should be avoided throughout pregnancy because the baby is at an increased risk for decompression sickness during this activity".[13]

Rounding out the activities to reconsider would include those that require a high degree of balance or that have a risk of falling and inducing trauma, like downhill skiing, skydiving, water skiing, kickball, or horseback riding.[14]

With these limitations aside, you can participate in most recreational activities. Exercising while pregnant by following these guidelines can actually keep your baby healthy, too. Research has shown prenatal exercise to have a favorable effect on babies in terms of their childhood body fat and neurological development all the way from birth to age 15.[15]

o Start slowly. Warm up; then do more demanding exercises; then cool down.

o Regular exercise, at least three times per week, is preferred to intermittent bursts of excessive activity. Doing a little bit of exercise in small bouts throughout the day is better than attempting your entire long exercise list only once a day. This will help you prevent overexerting yourself.

o Do all your exercises at a slow and controlled pace.

o Exercise on a firm, gentle surface, like a carpeted floor. Avoid surfaces that are too hard or too soft. Too hard will be uncomfortable for you on the side that is on the ground. Too soft and you sink and sag into the surface, letting your ligaments get overstretched where you're lacking support.

o Non weight-bearing are preferred over weight-bearing exercises.

▪ Evidence suggests that weight-bearing exercise use up your oxygen reserve more than non weight-bearing exercise.[16]

- Weight-bearing is just that. You are bearing weight through the chain of joints that makes up your skeleton. As your baby grows, the pressure on these joints is magnified. This pressure often creates discomfort during pregnancy sooner than non weight-bearing exercise.
- Non or reduced weight-bearing ideas: cycling, swimming, water walking, prenatal pool classes.
- Weight-bearing: walking, running, aerobics classes. If you are used to doing these activities well before becoming pregnant, carry on as tolerated. Modify to lesser intensity as needed due to pain or fatigue—like taking a walk instead of jogging.
- If weight-bearing feels good, do it. Some exercise is better than no exercise. My intention here is to spell out which type causes more joint pressure. In no way am I attempting to discourage weight-bearing options.

o Breathing and heart rate should be your normal rates, prior to starting your exercise. The staff you're getting to know really well at your OBGYN's office is checking both at the beginning of each checkup. Wvrite down your baseline numbers during your next visit, so you have that as a reference point. If any of the warning signs outlined for when to stop exercise occur, count your breaths and heartbeats per minute.

- Use the Talk Test as your basic guide. Recent guidelines actually no longer focus on where your numbers are. Your heart rate may not rise with exercise the same way it did before pregnancy. More important than numbers is how you feel. If you can comfortably carry on a conversation while exercising, it's unlikely that you're overexerting yourself.[17]

o   Don't overexert yourself at the beginning. Getting burned out or quitting early lacks staying power for an exercise program.

o   Before starting, have a snack. When you exercise during pregnancy, your body needs an additional 200 calories for itself and an additional 300 calories for the baby.

o   Stay hydrated! To calculate your needed daily fluid intake, take your weight and divide it by 2. For example: 170 ÷ 2 = 85. You need 85 ounces of water for your normal daily activities plus additional fluids on days when you perform more strenuous exercise or sweat a lot. Water is best, but other beverages count toward your daily total.

   ▪   Dehydration could make you feel thirsty and give you a dry, sticky mouth, or make you sleepy or dizzy. If you notice you haven't needed your usual extra trips to the bathroom, or have a headache, these are also warning signs to increase your fluids.

o   Pre-pregnancy routines can be resumed gradually after six to eight weeks postpartum.

WARNING SIGNS TO STOP EXERCISING

Warning signs are pain, especially pubic pain; feeling dizzy or faint; feeling breathless; pounding, racing, or irregular heartbeat; absence of fetal movement; uterine contractions; or vaginal bleeding.[18]

If you feel any pain, dizziness, or shortness of breath, stop and rest! If you feel better, resume exercise at a slower pace. Do not exercise to exhaustion. Discontinue exercise for the remaining duration of the pregnancy if you continue to experience the warning signs listed above, and definitely take notes on what you were doing when you felt this way.

Call your doctor if the symptoms do not let up after you have adequately rested.

You're a Fit Mom!

Women that are more physically fit generally have less back pain during pregnancy.[19] Even if you don't do any exercise yet, you're looking for answers by reading this book. You've taken the first step toward physical fitness, less back pain, and a happier pregnancy (and life after pregnancy!).

What I did during pregnancy and still do now are outlined below. Try these on for size, and add little daily bouts of your favorites to keep yourself moving.

EXERCISE

Exercising during a normal pregnancy typically doesn't cause any stress on your baby. Worries of exercise harming you or your growing baby have lessened in recent years. As such, the restrictions have lessened, too.

This is great! You may continue dancing, exercise classes, or specific athletic training during your pregnancy. If you wish to continue these, keep your family doc and OB in the loop to OK the program and supervise if necessary.[20]

Dedicated exercisers have asked me the most questions about the aerobic activities outlined below. I'll go through ways to continue the exercises you love for as long as possible during your pregnancy.

It's important to mention the idea of "good" pain and "bad" pain. Sharp or persistent pain means something is too tight or weak in that area to continue doing things the way you're doing them. Mild muscle soreness for up to 48 hours following an exercise session is considered normal.[21]

The biggest rule of thumb is to listen to your body. Pain is the stimulus that is telling your body to change what you're doing.

Rotating or Twisting Movements

I include the open-book and lower-trunk rotation exercises in the next chapter, which are safe, gentle stretches to do throughout your entire pregnancy. Moderate twisting would be fine throughout your pregnancy. Due to ligament laxity pre and postpartum, rigorous twisting during exercise should be done with caution.[22]

Prone Plank

This one is OK in the early to middle stages of pregnancy. If you choose to continue these in the third trimester, the increased pressure on your abdominal wall can contribute to diastasis recti or hernias that may not reveal themselves until postpartum.

Squatting

The coolest research article came out in 2018, "How to squat?"[23] I'll get right to the good stuff.

If your toes point forward, that is 0° of rotation. Rotating them out increases your angle of rotation. 0° and 42° were the most extreme angles observed when squatting and put the most strain on your hips and knees.

Avoid the extremes, and you'll avoid the pain and strain. Keep your toe-out angle wherever is comfortable between 0-42°. Everyone is different! That was the moral of the story, there's no picture of one perfect squat. Your best squat is different from my best squat.

This holds true during pregnancy. Change your typical set up if your hips or knees start hurting when you squat. Otherwise, stick to what your body knows and likes. If you have balance issues, being more front-heavy with the weight distribution of carrying the baby, hold on to something for support.

Dead Lifting

Lifting is OK to continue through weeks 22-30, depending on how fast your baby bump grows and how you feel. Use the same movement principles you would use if you were not pregnant: neutral spine, good ab muscle sequencing, and breathing patterns. If it sounds like I'm speaking a foreign language, and you weren't dead lifting before, now is not the time to introduce this tougher exercise.

If your body is well-trained or you are under the weekly care of a trainer or doctor, they can help find your desired weight to lift. If there is any strain on your pelvic floor, a big pull across your tummy, or any urine leakage, stop. You may need to decrease the weight you use each week. Otherwise, below is a standardized chart for lifting precautions.

	Intermittent Lifting		Repetitive Lifting	
WEEK OF GESTATION	Kilograms	Pounds	Kilograms	Pounds
20			>23 kg	>51 lbs
24			11-23 kg	24-51 lbs
30	>23 kg	>51 lbs		
40	<14 kg	<31 lbs	<11 kg	<24 lbs

American Medical Association Weight Limits for
Occupational Lifting During Pregnancy[24]

Are you carrying another child every day? Your body has muscle memory for this. Continue lifting them as long as it feels OK. My oldest was 21.5 months old when my second arrived, and I was carrying her until the end. She was about 25 pounds at that time. Every pregnancy is different, and the rules may not apply perfectly to you.

This chart was published to keep pregnant women safe at work, but these are good guidelines for an uncomplicated pregnancy for any day-to-day lifting in general.

Here's another good chart for all the data and metrics lovers out there. This contains a summary of the forces on your body from common activities, many of which I'll detail pregnancy considerations for below.

ACTIVITY	Peak Tibial Forces (x Body Weight)	Notes
Rowing Machine	0.9 ± 0.1	
Stationary Bicycling	1.0 - 1.5	Level 1-5; 60-90 rpm
Treadmill Walking	2.1 ± 0.2	1 to 3 miles per hour
Elliptical Level 11	2.2 ± 0.3	
Elliptical Level 1	2.3 ± 0.2	
Walking	2.5 - 2.8	Floor
Power Walking	2.8 ± 0.4	4 miles per hour on treadmill
Jogging	4.2 ± 0.2	5 miles per hour on treadmill

Peak Body Weight Forces of Activities[25]

Cycling Indoors

Cyclers: Want to continue using your bicycle? Sticking with your stationary bike while you're pregnant is great! The air temperature is controlled, and you're seated, so the risk for falling is quite low.

Additionally, it's less pounding on your body. At light to moderate resistance levels and 60-90 rpm (how fast you pedal), the body weight forces range from 1.0-1.5. So, it's just above the impact you feel standing still.

Here are some changes you could make to increase your cycling comfort as your belly grows:

o   Adjust the saddle position for your new comfortable angle.

o   Raise the handlebars and bring them closer to you to help you sit more upright, instead of straining your back to lean forward.

o   Dial back your intensity. It's normal to feel short of breath much faster.

Rowing Machine

A seated rower or "erg" rower is another good non-weight-bearing option, with forces on your body being around .9 body weight. This, of course, is only true when you use good movement patterns.[26] Pregnant rowers who experience limitations on knee-to-chest compression by their larger bellies may try to compensate by rotating the hips out, which places significantly more strain on the knees.

The fix: Avoid placing your feet too high on the footplate. Scoot them down as far as the machine allows. Put the strap right over your toes. That puts your knees lower and gives room for your baby to go between your knees. This will allow you to achieve good pressing power with your legs.

Your total motion, or how much you pivot, will be lessened now. Your belly will limit some of that movement, but that's normal and OK. Aim to pull the handle above your bump, hitting just below your breasts.

Kayaking

Kayaking is getting more and more popular every year, which is great! When kayaking pregnant, paddle below your normal intensity level. Borrow gear in a larger size to accommodate your belly.

Jumping Rope

The issue with jumping is that normal gravity is multiplied, placing more stress and strain on your body. Walking places a force of about 2.5x your body weight on you, and jogging on a treadmill at five miles per hour places a force of 4.2x your body weight. Jumping from a .45 meter height (18-inch box) is 5-7x your body weight into your joints and ligaments. The forces with jumping rope will fall closer to those of jogging.

If you're experienced in jogging and aerobics, the ACOG says you should be able to continue doing high-impact workouts safely. The biggest potential risks with jumping while pregnant are the uterus pounding down on the cervix, overstretching your ligaments, and the possibility of triggering contractions.[27]

RUNNING

Just yesterday I saw my very-pregnant neighbor walking the block with her husband. It brought back memories. I did my best to keep moving during the final weeks, too. In fact, the most popular way women try to self-induce labor is to walk.

Running is also safe during pregnancy. Many competitive, long-distance runners continue to run during their pregnancy. Many runners cut their training intensity to about half of their pre-pregnancy effort. Less than 4% of dedicated runners reported getting a running injury while pregnant.[28]

Are you a runner? If running is your passion, or your stress-relief, run on, sister. Healthy women that run deliver, on average, five to seven days sooner than non-runners. This may have some appeal!

My roommate from physical therapy school, Maureen, is an avid runner. Her goal was to run six miles every day until she was six months pregnant. At seven months, she lowered her mileage based on how she felt for that day. By the end, her pace was a slower, 14-minute mile. She was still running, and she had two healthy deliveries of ten-pound babies!

For her (and maybe you), running feels easier than walking because she'd trained her body to run. The longer step-lengths of walking caused pain. Try a walk/run combination. Do what feels better for your body if you're preparing for a pregnancy or you're in the middle of one!

If you need support, a running belt could be a good idea. Do a run without the belt, then with the belt. Do a run with the tape (covered later in the book) and stick with the option you like best. Many women who feel like their pregnant belly is just pulling down too much do prefer to use a belt to improve their comfort.

Pro Tip: If it feels like you're going to the bathroom a million times during the day, plan a route that puts you near a bathroom about every two miles.

Chapter 4 Key Points
- o   Exercise is generally good and OK to do while pregnant.
- o   Listen to your body. Pain is the stimulus that is telling your body to change.
- o   Snack before you exercise, and stay hydrated.
- o   Small, routine changes to the way you move during the day help more than pounding out an hour of exercise once a week.

CHAPTER FIVE

Exercise You Can Start in Your First Trimester

The Details

"What exercises can I do to prevent pain from happening?" As I was chatting with my pregnant friends (it always seems like there's a lot of those, right?), this was a question that came up a lot while their baby bump was still small.

This and Chapter 10 with the Kinesiology tape almost tie for the longest chapter. Read through these exercises now. Bookmark or dog-ear the page to reference later.

If you learn better by seeing someone do it first, check out my videos. I posted videos on <u>www.pregnancypainbook.com</u> for every exercise outlined here.

LOWER BACK STRETCHES

Prevention is the best medicine for lower back pain. These are my favorite tried and tested stretches to keep your back and body moving well during pregnancy. Do your favorites twice a day.

Most are done on your back, and you hold the stretch anywhere from five to thirty seconds, depending on how tight you are to start with. The final stretch is done lying on your side.

Remember: while flat on your back, stay in this position no more than five minutes due to vena cava compression in the third trimester (see Chapter 1). You may do these as long as you like, and you're feeling good, during the first and second trimesters.

Bed Stretches
Let your body go where it needs to comfortably stretch the most.

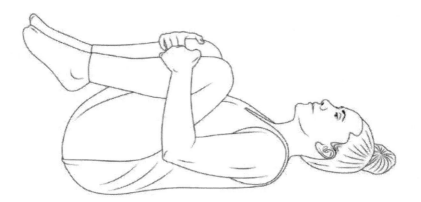

o **Double Knee to Chest**
   Lie on your back. Pull both knees to your shoulders. You may or may not feel your butt muscles gently stretching. The real beauty here is that it stretches the lowest portion of your lower back, that gets tight and compressed during pregnancy.
   Hold for 20 seconds.

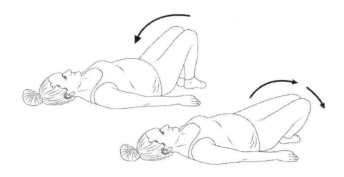

- **Lower Trunk Rotations**

  Lie on your back. With your knees bent, place feet together, and let your knees rock from side to side as far as you can comfortably. Repeat ten times.

  If rocking to one side increases back pain, do not rock to that side. For this exercise you rock to the "good" side(s) only.

- **Piriformis Stretch**

  There are two different ways to do this. Test both. Whichever is better for you, circle that one. That's the one for you. You will feel a comfortable stretch in your butt.

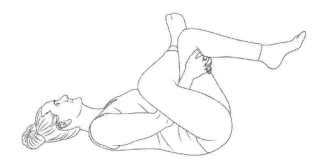

- **Option 1: Pull to stretch**

  Lie on your back. Place your ankle across your opposite bent knee. Pull your top knee toward the opposite shoulder. Hold for 20 seconds on each side.

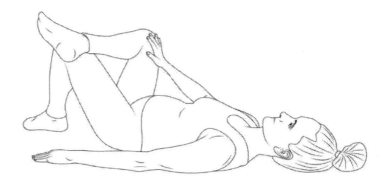

- **Option 2: Push to stretch**
  Lie on your back. Place your ankle across the bent knee. With your hand, push the top knee away from you.
  Hold for 20 seconds on each side.

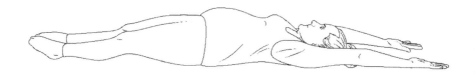

o **Trunk Elongation AKA "Get Taller" Stretch**
  Lie on your back with your legs flat. Reach your toes toward your footboard, or the foot end
  of your mattress. Squirm your hips around in a circle or side to side too. Push your head into the pillow. Reach your arms toward your headboard.

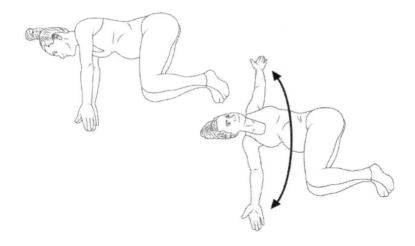

- **Open Book Stretch**

  Lie on your side with arms at a 90-degree angle from your body and your hands together. Rotate your body and pull the top arm away from the bottom arm, gently rotating the entire spine, as if your body was a book, and you open it up. Your nose should follow your hands. If you're really flexible, both of your shoulder blades will now be on the bed. If you're more stiff, stop before this creates any increase in pain.

  Return to start.

  It should take five seconds to open the book and five seconds to close the book.

  Repeat ten times each for the right and left sides. Like the trunk rotations, only do this on the side(s) that feel "good".

Try all of these tonight before you go to bed. Do them again in the morning. Listen to your body. If some feel like they're too easy and a waste of time, you probably have enough flexibility in that direction. If some feel like a good stretch, those are the ones to make time for. For me, the Open Books followed by the Piriformis Stretch's Pull Option are part of my secret recipe for keeping my back pain under control.

"What can I do if my pain happens at work or the store?"

Here's a great option for when you're not in bed.

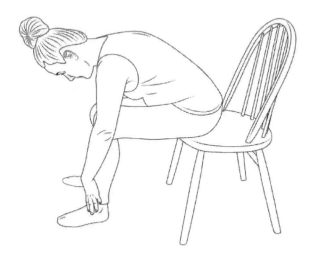

o **Seated Lower Back Stretch**
Sit in a chair. Open your hips and knees wide. Feet flat on the floor. Lean forward slightly at the hips keeping your back straight.
Count five down and five up.
Repeat five times.

The next time your back pain is higher than normal, open up to this page, and do the stretches that feel good! Circle those that help and do them most days of the week. You'll see a great improvement in your lower back.

SHOULDER AND NECK EXERCISES

Tight shoulders or neck? These exercises take away the strain to those areas. Your body is a tower, remember? Your shoulder blades are the base for your neck and shoulders. These are the most basic starting points to keeping the middle part of your tower in shape.

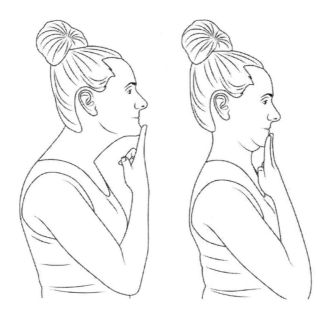

o **Chin Tuck**

Place your index finger on your forehead and push your head back, making a double chin. You should feel light pulling in the back of your neck and on the sides of your throat. Do them in your car, at traffic lights. Double chins are super cute, I know, but they should feel nice if this stretch becomes your new norm.

Hold for five seconds. Repeat ten times (or until the light turns green).

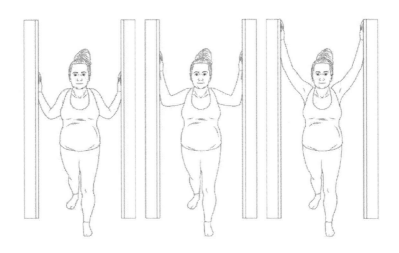

o **Chest Stretch in a Door**
   Stand in a door frame and place one hand on each side of the
   frame. Your fingers point up to the ceiling. Gently step one foot
   forward until you feel a stretch in the front of your chest, your
   pectorals. Keep your chest up and avoid letting your back arch a
   lot. If you feel any sharp pain in your shoulders or tingling in your
   hands, place your hands lower on the door frame. There are
   multiple angles to stretch your chest, and my picture covers your
   three major choices. Find the angle that feels best for you.
   Hold for 20 seconds.

ABDOMINAL AND PELVIC MUSCLE EXERCISES

Do you have back pain after doing anything for a prolonged amount of
time (maybe due to poor posture)? These exercises will help by
improving your sense of body-position awareness and the strength and
mobility of your lower back, pelvis, and hips.

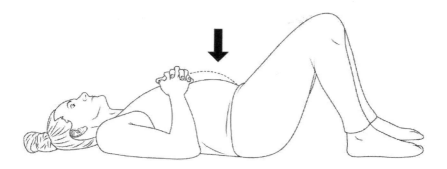

- **Abdominal Bracing AKA Posterior Pelvic Tilt AKA Transverse Abdominis Contraction**
  - **Phase 1: Lie on your back with your knees bent.**
    Tighten your stomach muscles and slightly pull your stomach down toward the bed or floor you're lying on. Your pelvis will tilt in such a way to smoosh your back flatter to the bed. Your shoulders should stay relaxed. If you're using "everything but the kitchen sink" to get this one done, you're doing it wrong. Another tip for this one: brace your abs "so it won't hurt if I punch you".
    Hold for five seconds. Repeat ten times.
  - **Phase 2: Change up the position!**
    - Sitting in the car
    - Sitting or standing at work
    - Before you lift something (good conditioning to get ready for lifting your bundle of joy!).

I want you to think about Abdominal Bracing as a new way of life, not as a chore or exercise. After you have mastered Phase 1, pay attention to what things in your day-to-day life give you twinges of pain in your low back. Pain is your body's best reminder, an early warning system!

The next time you start to get that twinge, brace your abs first. Eventually you'll retrain yourself to brace first and prevent the pain. Stick with it. It can take a few weeks to really make this a part of your normal movement through life.

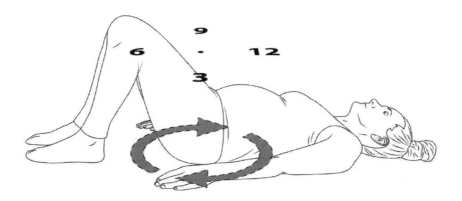

o **Pelvic Clocks**

These will help you isolate movement in your abs, back and pelvis to build awareness of the position of your spine with exercise and daily activities. This helps you tune in faster and correct painful activities.

Lie on your back with your knees bent. Paint an imaginary face of a clock on your lower abs. Your belly button is 12 o'clock. 6 o'clock is the top of your pubic bone. 3 and 9 o'clock are your hip bones.

- Gently rock your clock from 12 to 6 like an exaggerated pelvic tilt from the previous exercise. 10 times.
- Gently rock your clock from 3 to 9 (left to right). 10 times.

Move smoothly with your abs and pelvis, and keep your upper body relaxed. Your back will stay almost 100% in contact with the floor while you do these.

Do these once or twice daily, or whenever you need to stretch out your back.

Ta-Da! Now you're a real Shakira. And those hips don't lie.

o **Diastasis Recti Prevention and Reduction Exercises.**
  If you have a split in your abs, as described in Chapter 3, do these!
  ▪ **Prevent: Transverse Abdominal Breathing Exercise**
    This works the muscle just under the "six pack" ab muscle.
    Sit with your legs crossed. Breathe in and expand your belly.
    Breathe out and pull your belly button toward your spine as
    you exhale.
    Do 30-second bouts of this (five reps or so), five times per day.

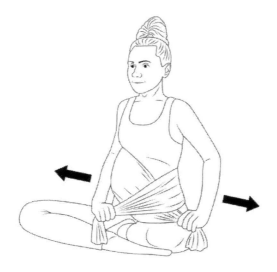

  ▪ **Reduce: Transverse Ab Exercise with Splint**
    For the splint you need a sheet, towel, dog leash, or stretching
    strap.
    Sit with your legs crossed. Wrap the splint around your lower
    back. Hold each end of the band in your hands and gently pull
    your arms apart. The band should crisscross together.
    Hold the abs together while you do the Abdominal Breathing
    Exercise.

KEGELS

A Kegel is a contraction of the muscles in your pelvic floor. Kegel exercises were developed in the late 1940s by an American gynecologist named Dr. Kegel. He developed these as a non-surgical way to help women prevent urine leakage.

Doing Kegels now will help keep your pelvic muscles in shape. Keeping the muscles around your vagina tight can lessen pre- or post-partum issues that are common with bladder leakage and help keep things fine-tuned for intimacy.[29]

Your pelvic floor is made up of several layers of tissue. There are two distinct muscle layers, on the other side of your vaginal opening, that you cannot see. Their job is to control the stream of urine, among a few other jobs.

When you carry and deliver a baby, the muscles in your pelvic floor get stretched more than normal and are often weakened. If you've had a previous delivery where a vacuum or forceps were needed, or you had any tearing, weakness is more likely.

Dribbling pee is no fun. Studies show you can make big improvements in this by training these muscles. Some can even *prevent* incontinence during pregnancy and after delivery.[30]

A basic Kegel program is appropriate for most people.

Kegels don't fix everything and occasionally doing Kegels could make your issue worse, if you're not ready for them. While Kegel exercises seem to be the go-to exercise for any issues in this area, many specialists argue that the opposite should be done in those cases. In this case, reverse Kegels come first.

The reason is that not everybody has a weak pelvic floor, but those muscles can actually be overactive. For the purpose of the book, most of you can jump right into the program below.

If you try a Kegel and it hurts, that means you should see a specialist for advice and personal help before you start this part of the exercise program. They'll figure out the source of your pain and start with those reverse Kegels, which are focused on relaxation of the muscles.

Identify the muscle gently first. Think about when you're sitting on the toilet, peeing. And you have to stop the pee mid-stream for whatever reason. Do this motion now. You should feel the muscles around the opening of your vagina tighten. You just did a Kegel!

Here's a basic at-home self-test for Kegels, to make sure you're doing them right. Finger Test: Put one finger in your vagina. Your muscles should grab and pull inward.

Additionally, you can look at the perineum, the area between your vagina and anus, with a mirror. You should see an "anal wink" and "clitoral nod" if correct, and no butt squeeze.

You should be able to perform these in a seated position without anyone noticing. You shouldn't see any other body movement; glute muscle contractions will make your body move up and down, so this is another good test.

The pelvic floor muscles are small and thin, so you're not going to see a lot of movement. You just have to make sure you're doing it right. For example, some women bear down onto the pelvic floor instead of drawing in and upward. Avoid straining or holding your breath with these. You should be able to talk and breathe normally.

A Kegel includes the contraction *and* full relaxation, or muscle returning to its relaxed state. Some people can feel the muscle letting go, others cannot.

A basic and well-rounded Kegel program includes ten each of both long holds and quick flicks, three separate times per day.

- o **Long Holds**: Tighten the pelvic floor and hold for up to ten seconds, rest for up to ten seconds. Repeat.
- o **Quick Flicks**: Tighten the pelvic floor and quickly release. Hold for one second, rest for two seconds. Repeat.

Use imagery to help. Pretend the pelvic floor is an elevator. At rest it is on the ground floor. Tighten a little to take it to the first floor, a moderate amount to the second floor, and all the way tight for the penthouse. Then slowly release in small amounts to come back down. This one's my favorite; you can really focus on controlling your muscles.

Just like other exercises, you should build up your stamina, so you don't get too sore too fast. You'll probably need to build up your long-hold strength before you can do ten seconds ten times. Avoid using extra muscles in the area, like the bigger glute muscles. Between sets, rest for an equal amount of time as the hold.

These are important, ladies.

Anyone watch Sex in the City? Every time I hear the word Kegel, I can hear Samantha Jones scrunching her nose and saying, "I'm doing mine right now." And I do a set until my muscles get tired or I get distracted.

Do Kegels anytime you're waiting for a traffic light to turn green, anytime the intro to the show you're binge-watching comes on, anytime you sneeze or cough, and anytime someone says the word Kegel!

Do Kegels every time you think of it. This will help you get to your three-times-per-day target.

STRENGTHENING FROM HOME

These are the top exercises to safely get stronger through your pregnancy. As a bonus, these muscles are the ones you need to carry your baby!

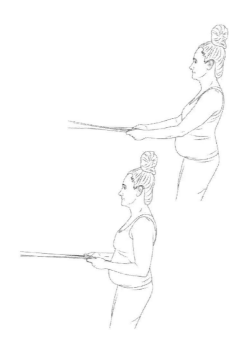

o **Shoulder Blade Pinch and Rows**
Pinch your shoulder blades together and down, toward your back pockets. Don't let your elbows stick out past your backside. Hold for five seconds. Repeat ten times.
To advance: Anchor a stretchy resistance band in a door, hold the band at its ends, and slowly pull back.

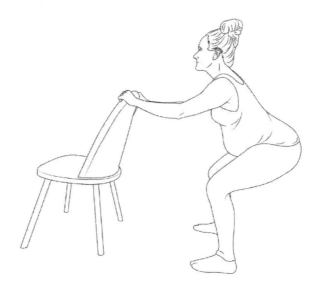

- **Modified Squats AKA "Thighs of Steel" ;)**

  If you wish to use squatting for labor, these are a must. If you want to protect your back with all the bending you're going to do when your tummy is too big, these are a must. If you want to pick your baby up from the crib without your back hurting, these are also a must. Live that squat life.

  Stand with your feet shoulder-width apart, or wider. Face a counter-top or hold on to the back of a chair. Slowly bend your knees and reach back with your butt as far as you comfortably can. You should always be able to see your toes. Keep your back straight. Slowly return to standing. If you have knee problems, do a mini squat as far down as you can bend your knees without turning your knee pain on too much.

  Hold for five seconds, 10 to 20 times.

  These are great to sprinkle in throughout the day. Throw in a set of ten when you sit down after returning from a bathroom break. I like to do a squat hold while I watch the microwave timer count down for my lunch.

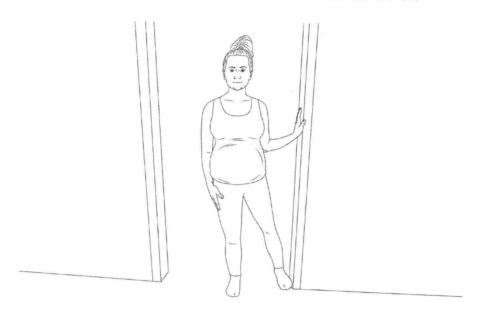

o **Standing Leg Side Raise AKA Hip Abduction**
Stand straight up in a door frame. Hold the door frame for balance.
Slowly kick one leg out to the side about eight inches and stop
when your foot meets the frame.

Make sure you keep your right and left hips at an equal height and
avoid hiking one up toward your ear.

Work up your long hold times to one minute on the right and one
minute on the left.

For me, doing this exercise most nights of the week while I brush
my teeth really helps keep my back strong. This strengthens the
gluteus medius, which is one of the most important muscles in your
lower body. I brush my top teeth while I do my right leg, then
brush my bottom teeth while I do my left leg. It's not a chore but
my new night routine, and it has really helped me.

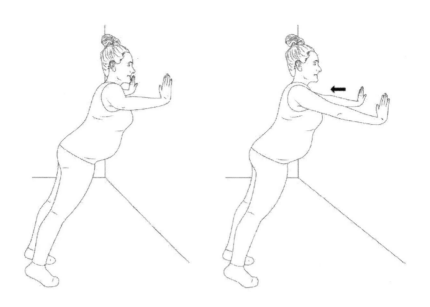

o **Wall Push Ups**

Stand facing a wall, a couple feet away from the wall. Place your arms out in front of you with your elbows straight. Your hands will touch the wall, at eye-level.

Next, bend your elbows slowly to bring your chest closer to the wall in a "push up" position. Then push your body away from the wall. Keep your chin tucked into your chest the whole time.

Repeat 10 to 20 times.

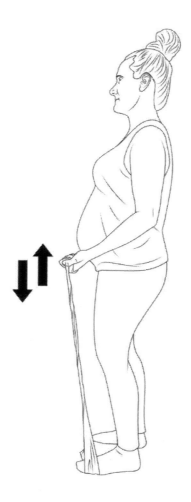

o **Bicep Curls**

In a standing position, place your feet shoulder width apart. Arms are at your sides. Bend your elbows all the way up, then straighten your arms all the way down. Keep your palms facing inward the entire time. Do this slowly up and slowly down.

Repeat 20 times.

Add weights. If your resistance band is long enough, step on the band as pictured. If you have hand weights, or an object that weighs a few pounds, use that.

POOL EXERCISE

Do you or a friend have a pool, or do you want to check out a pre-natal exercise class? Keep in mind the general exercise guidelines outlined previously.

Exercising in a pool when you're pregnant is great! It feels like you're walking on the moon, without gravity pulling down your growing body.

Pool exercise helps with swelling, blood pressure, heart rate, and even digestion. Getting in the pool also improves joint pain and grows muscle strength.

Here are the things you need to know to exercise safely in a pool:
- A good depth is four feet deep. Too much more and you'll lose control of your body.
- Start easy. Do 40 minutes then stop. Wait to see how your body responds.
- Avoid too hot or too cold water or air temperature.
  - Therapy pools set their target temperature between 90-94 degrees Fahrenheit.
  - When you're pregnant, it is easy to get overheated—therefore, cooler water is preferred. Also, since it's so easy to get sweaty when you're pregnant, the cooler water usually feels better.
  - A study in Australia found that water temperature up to 91.4F (33C) is safe for moderate-intensity aerobic pool exercise during pregnancy. Cooler water down to 82.4F (28C) was also found to be safe.[31] If the water is colder than that, listen to your body.

- Keep in mind that air temperature has a major effect on how the pool temperature feels. Exiting a warm indoor pool to a cold locker room or to get back into your car can be extreme. If your body doesn't handle extreme temperature changes well, schedule your pool time on milder days.
  - Avoid indoor pool fumes for excessive periods of time. Prolonged exposure to Chlorine fumes could make you feel ill.[32] Moderate, routine exposure followed by fresh air is best.
  - Monitor your blood pressure and any light-headedness before you get in, during, and when you get out of the water if you have any concerns about how your body will react.
  - Take a water bottle to keep poolside. In a pool, your body actually sweats, but you don't actively see the perspiration. Stay hydrated to account for this.
    - I was a pool Physical Therapist for three years. When I first started, I would exit the pool and have a headache for hours. I drank an extra coffee, but that didn't fix the issue. Turns out, I was dehydrated. Keeping water on the side of the pool was the fix.

Below is the backbone of the pool exercises I share with all my patients who want to use the pool. I still do some of these things when I take the kids swimming—that is, *if* the water is warm enough for me to get in!

Pool Exercise Program
Start with 10 reps, then 20, then 30 of each.

If any of these make your pain worse, back off of the exercises for two days.

o **Feet on the Ground (Standing Exercises)**
  - **Forward Walking**- three laps down and back slowly each time. Keep abdominals tight the whole time. Small steps to turn at the end of the lane.
  - **Backward Walking**- three laps down and back slowly each time. Keep abdominals tight the whole time. Small steps to turn at the end of the lane.
  - **Sideways Walking**- three laps down and back slowly each time. Keep abdominals tight the whole time. Face the same way down and back.
  - **Arms Raises 3 Ways**-
    - Start with your arms floating on the surface of the water in front of you. With your palms facing down, push hands down to your stomach. Raise them back up slowly.
    - With your arms floating on the surface of the water, out to your sides, turn your palms facing down. Push your arms down under the water until your hands touch the sides of your legs, then raise them back up slowly.
    - With your arms floating on the surface of the water, out to your sides, turn your palms facing in. Bring your arms together until your hands clap, then slowly open your arms back up again.
  - **Row the Boat**- With your arms in front of you, pull back imaginary paddles and row the boat. Squeeze your shoulder blades together, then return your arms to the reaching position.

- **Holding the Side of the Pool**
    - **Leg Raises 3 ways-** Forward, side, back. Leg straight, abs tight, raise your leg 12 inches in each direction.
    - **Heel and Toe Raises-** Rise up to toes, count to five. Rock back to heels, count to five. Do not let your butt stick out.
    - **Mini Squats-** Bend knees and reach butt back, stay in your in pain free motion, or squat as far as you can while keeping your head above water.
    - **Calf Stretches-** Place one foot close to the wall of the pool, and step back about three feet with the other foot. Plant the heel of the back foot on the ground. Gently lunge forward until you can feel the muscle in your lower leg stretching on the leg that is back. Hold each side for one minute.
- **Deep Water-** Loop two noodles or floatation belt around you.
    - **Bike** (pedal like you're riding a bike) for five minutes, keeping legs underneath you.

Check out www.pregnancypainbook.com for these pool exercises, and all the land exercises, too.

Chapter 5 Key Points
- Do ten Kegels right now!
- Dog-ear or mark this Chapter. Exercising at home is excellent preventative medicine for back pain that won't quit.
- If it feels good, do more of it. If it hurts, stop that exercise for the day.
- The pool is a weightless exercise zone; enjoy it! Just make sure you take a water bottle to keep poolside, and don't get overheated.

CHAPTER SIX

MEDICAL AND NATURAL TREATMENTS YOU CAN START IN THE FIRST TRIMESTER

The foot bone's connected to the leg bone… the leg bone's connected to the knee bone.

Or try this variation:
The car tire's connected to the car bearing… the car bearing's connected to the car axle.

You have your car serviced every 10,000 miles. You put air in the tire when it's flat. Your body is your ride for life. Take care of it. Here are some tips on self-maintenance or the professionals you should take your body to if your tire is a little low, or if it's making a funny sound as it goes down the road.

PHYSICAL THERAPY

If there is a kink somewhere in your body, or the air in your tire is low on one side, it'll only worsen with time. Later, the issues will spread to the next body part over. The ankle bone is connected to the leg bone, after all.

Think of it like that 10,000 mile tune up. If your car tire is getting flat, don't you think that another warning light or weird noise is going to start? You bet! It's only a matter of time. As such, pain is your body's warning system that something's going on.

Physical Therapists (PTs) are Body Mechanics. We watch people move.

All.
The.
Time.

You people-watch for fun. We can't turn off our movement analyzing, even at the beach, the store, or when we watch our favorite show! We are really good at finding a hitch in your giddy-up (AKA, something weird in your movement) and knowing what to do to fix it.

Most of the pregnant patients that I help are already in their third trimester, and they've had pain for months. Months!! If there is trouble brewing, get help as soon as possible.

Most states in the United States have direct access to physical therapy. This means you can hop on the internet and search "physical therapy near me" or "PT for pregnancy pain" and schedule an appointment to get to the root of your issues right away at a place with excellent reviews.

Any "change in status" is enough to open a new door to PT. This could be a new pregnancy and you're having back pain, sudden carpal tunnel while typing, getting into a car accident, or missing the bottom step and straining your back. We're talking real life, here.

When I was pregnant with #2, I fell *up* the stairs. I was in socked feet, on hardwood floors, at my in-law's house. I thought my mother-in-law would faint. Basically, anything awful that happens in real life is made one hundred times worse when you're pregnant! The next day I spoke to my PT and they got me on a plan to help with my new strain.

Sit down and make sure you're OK. Dust yourself off. Do as much of your normal routine as you can for the next 48 hours. If you're jammed up and can't un-jam yourself, that's when you ask for help.

Other day-to-day things that PT helps with are having pain so bad you can't use your favorite machine at the gym, or even having pain walking from your car into work. I've even seen a pregnant patient who threw her back out from sneezing! Relaxin does some serious work in our bodies to keep things loose for your growing baby—sometimes too loose!

A Good PT:
- Sees no more than two clients per hour. You want their attention.
- Uses their specialized, hands-on skills every day. They routinely perform Grade 5 Mobilizations, AKA Manipulations. This is a fast, small change made exactly where the kink is in your hose. After that, your joints and muscles move better. They'll get right to the root of your problem, and adapt their pressure knowing that you're pregnant.

Getting PT early can make the remainder of your pregnancy less of a "pain in the butt" so you can focus more on the joy.

Pro Tip: Always tell your medical providers that you're pregnant, even if your baby belly isn't showing yet. Tell them, even if you haven't announced your pregnancy to your job or your hundreds of Facebook friends. It could affect which treatments they use, as they will alter their practice to what is safest for you and your baby.

73

MASSAGE

Tight muscles develop due to the changing pulls on your back, arms, and legs when you're pregnant. Awkward work or home postures make muscles work too hard. Fix your posture where possible.

Getting a massage is good for the knots that come back despite the best posture set-up. Having a massage during your pregnancy, especially during the final months, can help with muscle tension, headaches, stress, and sleep.[33]

Stick with a massage therapist who has experience working with pregnant women. Many states require therapists to be certified in prenatal massage. If you have a high-risk pregnancy, tell the therapist exactly what's going on. It may be safer to wait until after the baby arrives.

Free Massages

Massage schools always need pregnant "clients" to work on for their certification. Hop online and search for "massage school". Find out where the closest one is. They should have open hours to get clients in each month. Many times, you can get these for free!

What to Avoid

Avoid your feet and ankles when getting a massage by someone you love. Stimulating the inside or outside of your ankles can turn on the reflex to your uterus and ovaries due to pressure points in these areas. This could trigger uterine contractions or cause cervical softening.

Some very pregnant women seek out massages to their feet to start labor if they are overdue. Does this always work? No. Could it work? In theory, yes. Play it safe and say, "No Thanks" to their offer, or find a professional. Unless of course you are past your due date, then the choice is yours.

HEAT OR ICE?

Ten to fifteen minutes of heat or ice can help soothe your sore muscles and joints. Heat relaxes. Ice calms inflammation.

"-itis" means inflammation, as seen in burs*itis,* tendon*itis,* and arthr*itis.* When something has inflammation or feels swollen, it is irritated. Your body sends extra blood flow to the area to help it heal. When too much extra blood flow hangs around, it becomes a problem, and makes you feel sore.

Heat increases blood flow to the area and does not help to decrease inflammation. It can also increase the flexibility of tissues.

Heat could feel good in the form of a warm shower to relax sore muscles, or a heating pad across your shoulders. Never use heat before you exercise, due to the extra movement in your ligaments when you are pregnant. The total increase in your flexibility can set you up to over-stretch and get hurt.

Ice helps to decrease inflammation and can really help reduce pain. Ice constricts or shrinks blood vessels, temporarily reducing the "-itis" to the area. After you put the ice away, the blood vessels return to their normal plumpness. A fresh flow of blood enters the area, flushing out the soreness chemicals.

Ice also slows down the signals that nerves send. If your nerve mutes the signal it sends to the brain, it takes the edge off of how loud your pain or aching joint is. Since taking nonsteroidal anti-inflammatory drugs (NSAIDs) is discouraged during pregnancy, ice is your first, best, and most natural choice to calm inflammation.

Before, during, and after my pregnancies I would often take a big reusable ice pack to bed with me. I would lie on it for ten minutes. I usually fell asleep. No big deal! When you wake up, throw the ice pack on the floor. When you get up the next day, put the ice pack in the freezer so it'll be cold again for the next time.

You can even do some of your exercises, like double knees to chest or lower trunk rotations, while you're lying on ice. It doesn't turn you into an ice sculpture; you can still move. I would even roll on to my side, lay it over my side, and let it drape over my back. This calmed down my sore back without medicine.

Ice is nice!

Chapter 6 Key Points
- o Anything dramatic that happens in real life is made one hundred times worse when you're pregnant.
- o Add a good Physical Therapist to your team, early on.
- o Call a local massage school about a free pregnancy massage.
- o Ice, Ice, Baby. Ten to fifteen minutes of heat or ice can help quiet your sore spots.
- o Do ten Kegels right now.

CHAPTER SEVEN

KEEP YOUR BLOOD FLOWING IN THE SECOND TRIMESTER

"She was nearly fainting: indeed, she wished she could really faint, but faints don't come for the asking." ~C.S. Lewis, *The Chronicles of Narnia: The Silver Chair*

Fainting in books gives dramatic effect. Fainting in real life, while you're pregnant, does too! Let's not add any more drama than needed.

BLOOD FLOW AND THE VENA CAVA

Compression on your important blood vessels can start in the fourth month of pregnancy. Prolonged standing in one place or lying on your back causes this to occur most often.

As mentioned in Chapter 1, the inferior vena cava is the vein smooshed by your uterus in those positions. Its job is to get blood from your legs to your heart, so this smooshing is definitely not good.

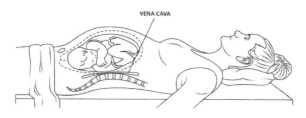

Vena cava syndrome

Compression can lead to placental separation—meaning less oxygen and nutrients to your baby and a decrease in kidney function for you. This compression can make you feel lightheaded or dizzy. You may actually pass out due to a quick drop in your blood pressure.

If you've been standing or lying on your back for a long time and just feel yucky, stand up slowly, then get moving! Keep that blood flowing. Heavy bleeding is another warning sign, after laying on your back or standing, that something is wrong.

After the fourth month of pregnancy, avoid lying on your back for more than five minutes. To lay on your back to give the sides of your hips a rest, or to do a brief exercise, roll up a hand towel or use a pillow and place it under your *right* hip, to elevate that side by at least four to five inches.

This will roll your uterus off of that vein and take the stress off your heart to pump the blood evenly through your body.[34]

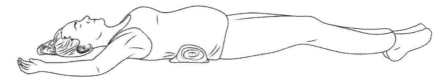

To prevent vena cava compression, if you lay on your back, use a towel roll to elevate your right hip at least four to five inches.

POSITIONAL LOW BLOOD PRESSURE AND FAINTING

AKA Orthostatic hypotension. This is a form of low blood pressure that you feel when you suddenly go from lying or sitting to a standing position. Essentially, your body can't keep up with pumping the blood to get to your brain now that it suddenly has to go uphill, against gravity.

How Does it Make You Feel?

With these quick changes in position, you could feel dizzy, lightheaded, or even faint. Dizziness is quite common during pregnancy, however, fainting does not happen to everyone.

Does fainting sound like fun? It's not! I have low blood pressure. I fainted when I was in the eighth grade. I was in Tech Ed class, watching our teacher make the sample project.

We were probably sitting for ten minutes. When I went to stand up, my vision went dark and the next thing I remember is waking up and being helped into a wheelchair. I'd slid from the classroom stool onto the ground. I got pushed in that wheelchair through seventh grade lunch. Can it get any more embarrassing than that?

Yes, it can: fainting when you're pregnant. If you've had low blood pressure before, now, or have ever had times when you feel dizzy, you should let your family and co-workers know. My mistake was that I stood up too fast. Always get up from lying or sitting positions slowly.

Fainting can happen if your brain temporarily doesn't get enough blood, causing you to go lights-out and lose consciousness briefly. If this happens, especially more than once, tell the doc.

What to Do If You or Someone Else Faints

If you feel faint, lie or sit down. If you're sitting, bring your head down between your knees, so the blood doesn't have to fight gravity to get to your brain.

If someone actually faints, assuming that you/they were not injured as they fainted, raise the person's legs above the level of their heart if possible. To do this, lay them on a couch and prop all the backrest cushions under their legs, or lay them on the floor and put their feet on the seat of a chair.

Help the person get up slowly, once they come to. If the person doesn't regain consciousness after one minute, call 911, as this could be a more serious case.[35]

WHAT NOT TO DO

Don't Bear Down
Bearing down can cause too much pressure on your uterus and pelvic floor muscles. Keeping your face and jaw relaxed can help with this when you're on the toilet or doing harder work. Holding your breath can cause you to unintentionally bear down.

If having a bowel movement is causing you too much strain, look into a Squatty Potty. This is a stool that lives at the base of your toilet. Your feet rest on it, thus raising your knees above your hips. The idea is the squat position helps reduce the need to strain.

We got one halfway through my second pregnancy. It was actually the best thing ever for potty training #1. It was the perfect step stool. It won't be in the way for the family, and it makes your visits to the potty more efficient.

Don't Lie on Your Stomach
I've mentioned this before, but it bears repeating: from about the third month of pregnancy to delivery, avoid this position. Your growing baby is no longer protected by your pelvis. If you really need a break from

the positions you're allowed to use, there are Belly Down Pregnancy Pillows.

Don't Raise Your Butt Higher Than Your Chest

When you're lying face down, don't stick your butt in the air. For example, avoid the "downward dog" position.

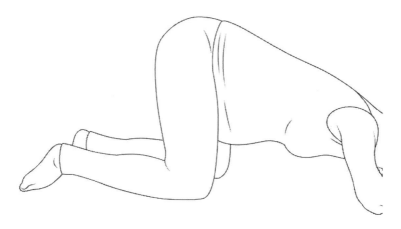

Avoid butt higher than chest

A rare but dangerous thing can happen during your second or third trimester, most especially in the six weeks after labor. If your butt is elevated above your head, your uterus can move up toward your head. When that happens, air can enter your bloodstream through the open placental site.

To review from the positions to avoid during intimacy, an air bubble in your vein is rare, but dangerous. These air bubbles can travel to other areas of your body, and could cause respiratory failure, a stroke or heart attack.

If you've had bleeding or other symptoms of placenta detachment occur during pregnancy, this position is a hard "no". *No one* should lie like this for six weeks after delivery.

Chapter 7 Key Points

- o Avoid lying on your stomach. Lying on your left side is best.
- o Don't raise your butt higher than your head.
- o It's easier to feel faint or lightheaded. Change positions slowly.
- o Do ten Kegels right now.

CHAPTER EIGHT

PRODUCTS TO BUY FOR YOURSELF IN THE SECOND TRIMESTER

Happy Second Trimester—the "honeymoon phase" for some. For many, the morning sickness has calmed, and your belly is growing into a cute but not unwieldy bump. Fluffing the nest for your baby-to-be can be super fun.

My next two Pro Tips come from a real pro. My patient Liz had four kids. She was about 30 when I worked with her for back pain, when her youngest was a few months old. It was great helping her move better while she tended to her flock. She also taught me some things.

LOTION

I'd heard a lot about cocoa butter for your pregnant belly. It was very easy to find. Some had better anti-stretch mark claims than others. Those lotions were OK, but the magic elixir here is lanolin. Liz didn't have any major stretch marks, and she was petite.

I started using this lanolin lotion as soon as my ticker started for the 13th week of pregnancy. I used it in the morning and at night after my shower. It really worked wonders and was cheaper than the expensive "best pregnancy lotions" advertised online.

Lanolin is a cruelty-free byproduct of wool. The only potential negative is that since lanolin comes from sheep, if you or someone in your house has a wool allergy, using this lotion could set off their symptoms. My husband got a stuffy nose if he was in the room when I put this on. I'm happy he stuck it out, because this stuff really worked.

Pro Tip: Don't forget "the girls." Put it on your breasts as soon as your old bras don't fit anymore. I made a mistake and stopped lotioning here after the baby came, for fear that the baby would eat the lotion.

Big Mistake. My milk was very slow to come in. But five days after labor, I woke up and my milk came all at once. Pow! And then came the stretch marks! The marks have faded with time but learn from my mistakes.

MATERNITY CLOTHES

Maternity Pants
Start with the pants.

Just buy the pants.

For my first pregnancy I was too proud to give up my pre-baby pants until the belly band that I bought to bridge the gap couldn't keep the gap closed anymore. A belly band looks like an oversized, fabric, headwrap-style headband that you use in place of a belt when you can't get your pants buttoned anymore.

Seemed like a good idea, and it did postpone buying pregnancy pants, but it was such a pain in the butt to get all the bells and whistles back in place after the frequent potty breaks! Save money and skip the belly band. It's important to be comfortable, especially in those early months when you're figuring out what this whole pregnancy thing is about.

Just buy the pants.

How many pairs of pants do you need? Now that I don't need pregnancy pants anymore, of course I made a friend that works at the maternity clothing store. For your first round of pregnancy clothes, my expert Jessica recommends one to two pairs each of jeans, work pants, and leggings/lounge pants.

Pregnancy/Maternity pants really are the best. No buttons. No zippers. Just slide 'em up. They are so comfy that my husband T.J. was jealous when an eating holiday came around, and he couldn't join me with the stretchy-waisted pants. I had two Thanksgivings in pregnancy pants.

The pants were a little too comfortable. T.J. had to pry them away from me when it was time to go back to work eight weeks after each baby arrived. They were so comfortable! I was attached to them, and I swore you couldn't tell they weren't "regular" pants. A new chapter was underway, though, and I rotated the pants with zippers back into my life.

Secret confession: When I found out we were having #2, I couldn't wait to bust them back out.

Maternity Bras

If you can wear a bra without the underwire, do that. The lack in rigidity of the wire gives you more flexibility to grow into it.

If you can, go for a flexible sizing option (i.e. Small/Medium/Large/XL vs 34B or 36DD) due to the same idea of being more a "one size fits most" than molded for a specific shape.

Pro Tip: Get measured! If you feel like you need the support that you only find with an underwire, the next big tip is to go get measured.

Brand name mall stores such as Victoria Secret and Hanes offer complimentary measuring.

Buy a bra where the connector hooks in the back have room to grow; today they are on the closest set of hooks, and you can use the farther-out hooks later. This will minimize the need for bra hook extenders, but those are a nice option too, to get more mileage out of your gear.

Maternity Underwear

Like finding a pair of jeans that fit just right, every booty has its own shape and fit—pregnant or not. Some of my friends never needed new undies during their pregnancies, but I did.

If you can't try on the underwear you think will fit, buy one pack of maternity underwear and one pack of your normal underwear that is two sizes bigger than you usually buy. It's literally 50/50 whether you will find the maternity underwear or the larger regular underwear the best fit for the way your body is shaped. Once you find a winner, get enough pairs to get you from one laundry day to the next.

Maternity Shirts

I listed shirts last, because not everyone buys these. You can either go with longer regular shirts or grab a few maternity shirts for a more fitted look. Option three here is to purchase nursing shirts instead. They are flowy and work with your pregnant belly, and you can get more wear out of these when the page turns to breast feeding.

MATERNITY BRACE

A maternity brace is a somewhat stretchy back brace designed to accommodate your pregnant belly. With your ligaments and muscles being overstretched on your backside, a little extra outer support can help relieve the pressure.

Will it help? Yes! Some are basic bands that rest over the top of your hips and hug your lower back. Some have an extra support strap that goes up and around your belly. I found a basic model, and it helped my pain during my second and third trimesters.

There are dozens of maternity support belt options out there, some of which include a top strap. Sizing is typically pretty accurate. Have your partner or a friend use a seamstress tape measure around your belly.

Getting the brace to fit correctly is critical. I liked wearing mine on top of an undershirt, with a top shirt over it. The brace should be snug but comfortable when you're standing. They work best when you are standing and walking and tend to get bunched up when you sit. If it bunches when you sit, give your skin time to breathe by taking a break from the brace when you'll be sitting for a while.

Refer back to the posture section in Chapter 1, and use the exterior support of a good chair.

Deep indents or impressions on your skin after removing the brace means you have the brace on too tight. Wear it looser next time.

Chapter 8 Key Points
- o   Try lanolin lotion.
- o   Score your maternity pants sooner rather than later.
- o   Get a maternity support belt if you are having lower back pain.
- o   Do ten Kegels right now.

CHAPTER NINE

PRODUCTS YOU NEED ON YOUR BABY REGISTRY TO REDUCE YOUR PAIN AND STRESS

Here is the top gear that you *need* in order to protect your body during "The Baby Years." This gear is listed in no particular order. They are all very, very useful things available at most places where you can set up a baby registry.

Do you need a registry? Yes! From the lips of my mother-in-law (a veteran baby shower hostess and attendee): "Things have changed since I've had babies. I want to get something useful, and I hate giving gift cards". Friends and family want their gifts to help, and they may need the guidance of your wish list.

You most definitely need a registry. And if someone asks where you're registered, graciously answer their question and let them be as generous as they are inclined to be. Keep a stash of thank you notes on hand. A six- to eight-pack of blank-on-the-inside note cards from the dollar store are my jam.

ERGO CARRIER OR SLING

Ergo Carrier vs Sling. An ergo carrier is like a baby backpack worn like a kangaroo in front of you. They have adjustable straps to snug the baby in tight. Follow the guidelines on the exact type you get when the baby is big enough. I waited until they had some head control.

Personally, I loved my carrier. I tried a sling, but I am a motor moron with new gadgets. I did not stick with it to figure out how to wrap up myself with the baby. If you have a friend that swears by one, have them help you practice using theirs with a baby doll, or their baby. Seriously.

Also, if you get one set up correctly, but when you use it your back or neck really hurt, try to adjust it. It could also be a sign that that particular carrier is not right for *you*.

Pro Tip: While we're on the subject of baby dolls, here's how to fit a baby properly in a carrier. Put the baby doll in the carrier. Snug up the carrier straps until you can kiss the baby's head. Now you have the right fit. A very experienced salesman at the baby store where we dumped all of our "New Baby New Furniture" money taught us that one. I think he kept a doll in that aisle of the store just to show off.

It worked! We bought two carriers! One for Mom and one for Dad. The "best carrier with the most support" didn't fit my 6'5" husband correctly. If you're tall like my husband, the Maclaren Baby Carrier is what you want.

Do you really need a carrier or sling?

Honestly, I didn't use it much with Baby #1, but Baby #2 was in it and didn't mind being in it – all the time. If you plan to have more than one kid, get one. If you can work while you care for your baby, get one. Do you ever do two or more things at once? Get one.

BIG TICKET FURNITURE

Having babies is expensive! Here's a run-down of some of the more expensive baby gear and a few tips on which to prioritize.

Nursing Glider + Stool

What to look for:

- o Swivel. If you find a good chair that swivels all the way around, 360°, spring for that! Picture yourself gently rocking your baby. Your little angel falls asleep. Now you have the impossible task of walking them over to their crib and placing them in without waking them up. Do you know what one of the hardest parts is? Getting your tired body up out of the chair with grace. Having a chair that rotates or swivels makes this so much easier. We loved ours so much that we held on to it beyond the diaper years; it even made the move when we bought our first house.

- o Head support. Find a nursing glider, chair, or rocker that comes up high enough to support your and your partner's head. This is so important. If your head is tired, it's going to get stiff hunched forward when your muscles are just too tired to hold it up.

- o Footrest vs Gliding Ottoman. Footrest 100%. The gliding ottoman seems like it makes sense, and the stores usually stage the chair and ottoman together. If you can buy just the chair, get just the chair. Save your money on the ottoman and spend it on a sturdy footstool instead. There are "nursing stools" that you can register for. But just like anything marketed for "pregnancy" or "baby", you'll pay at least double for a comparable item that you can grab anywhere. Any footstool or ottoman that brings the floor to meet your feet works. If you have long legs, you may not even need a stool.

Crib + Dresser Set + Changing Table

Do *not* spend your whole paycheck on this furniture. This is my husband T.J.'s number one tip for expecting parents. Yes, new furniture looks good, and you can post cute pics on social media during the Nesting Phase. But do you have the budget to replace these things in five years?

Our babies used the rails of their not-cheap convertible crib bed frame as a teether! This was despite me spending even more money on Crib Rail Covers. They found all the exposed wood they could.

Ours converted from a crib, then to a toddler bed, and finally by adding an extra piece, to a full sized bed frame. And let me tell you, when they're in the full size bed from this "grow into it" "buy once, cry once" frame as an Elementary Schooler, they will be embarrassed about their beat-up furniture. #1 is asking when she can get new furniture. It's gonna be a while!

In hindsight, we should have taken the time to find a pre-loved set. The cost of a fresh coat of finish or paint would have been worth the money we saved. It would have saved the stress of our sweet angels chewing on and banging up the nicest furniture in the house too!

Later we could upgrade them to newer "big kid" furniture that they felt invested in choosing and thus responsible to care for as they grew up.

A few other notes on furniture. Find a low dresser that you can fit a 20-dollar diaper changing pad on top of. When the diaper years are over, the pad is easy to pitch. No need for a stand-alone "changing table".

Strangely enough, updating the dressers in our house may have kick-started my labor. Four days before my due date for #1, I was hard-core nesting.

Our guest room was transformed into the Baby's room. We had to empty and get rid of a tall dresser to make room for a low dresser. I was carrying drawers full of clothes. That night at one a.m. my contractions hit the magic number! Tuck that tip away for your final week; the final nesting has a purpose!

If you're going for a pre-loved crib, find out what the updated safety regulations are on spacing between slats, types of bumpers, etc. This goes for bassinets too. If you find a previously owned crib or bassinet, do an online search for recalls just to be sure it's OK. Safety first.

NURSING/FEEDING PILLOW

Not everyone breastfeeds. The pillow here is useful whether or not you plan to nurse. If you or someone gives the baby a bottle, you'll use a very similar set-up as you do with breastfeeding. A nursing pillow is perfect for bottle feeding, and breastfeeding. Get ready for milk mustaches on your little baby—they're the best!

A Boppy is the name brand for a nursing pillow. It's shaped like a horseshoe and hugs your body. I registered for one, but I didn't register for the extra cases (like a pillowcase but shaped like a horseshoe to specifically fit on this thing).

By the time Baby #2 arrived, I had acquired four Boppy pillows! I kept one in the chair I nursed in the most, in the actual nursery. I kept the second on the couch in front of the TV downstairs. The third lived at my parents' house—AKA our #1 babysitters. I kept the fourth at my husband's parents' house, where we visited regularly.

If we traveled for two or more nights, I packed my #1 Boppy. Really, don't leave home without it! You can try to prop pillows to do the same job, but they slide all over the place. Then you're left with a stiff back or shoulders because you're trying to be a frozen statue when your pillow falls and you don't want to disturb the baby you're trying to feed or rock to sleep.

Similar to the Boppy is the My Brest Friend nursing pillow. It has a strap that you secure around yourself, making for an easier transfer for the snoozing baby from your lap to their crib. Not sure which you'll like better? Register for one of each. Put them in different locations so you can always have support. Unsupported arms when feeding your baby equals sore muscles.

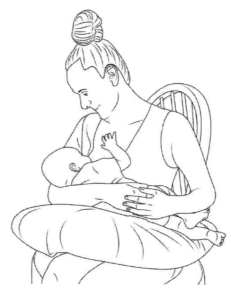

Nursing Posture

NURSING AND PUMPING GEAR

Not everyone breastfeeds. If you plan to breastfeed, here are the things I wish I knew. If you hit a wall with breastfeeding, as covered in a later Chapter, a lactation consultant will become an MVP. They're especially great during your baby's first weeks and every time they hit a growth spurt or change in routine.

Definitely get a pump with good reviews, and definitely check your insurance coverage. Many insurance companies now cover the cost of a pump. If so, get one ahead of time if you can, so you're not like me, running around town with an infant trying to get your last gear in place. I didn't think I would need a pump until I returned to work after my maternity leave.

On the contrary, pumps are very necessary from early-on. You'll want one, so you can start banking your milk.

One thing I don't think insurance pays for is extra valves. The funnel cups your breast, and there is a valve that connects the funnel to the bottle where you collect your "baby milk." Since you can buy "cow milk" at the store, "baby milk" is what our toddler called breast milk. It's what our kids still call it when we run into a hungry baby!

The valve is rubber and, like any rubber connector, can get loose or wear out after repeated use and cleaning. If you can see daylight through the straight part where the two sides of the valve come together, it's trash. Throw that sucker away. If an old valve makes the suction weak, it'll waste your time and yield less milk.

In addition to an electric pump, a one-sided hand pump can be helpful to have. You can use it for car rides out of town. They're also useful when the baby is sleeping through the night and you need to let off a little pressure.

Breast Milk = White Gold. It is exhausting, but it's totally worth every drop collected. Add six packs of extra breast pump valves to your registry list. They are specific to the brand of pump you want. If any arrive damaged, ask for your money back.

Pumping Bra

If you plan to stick with breastfeeding for a while, get two. They look like a strapless bra with a hole for each nipple to stick out of. They're totally hot.

Drops of milk can get rancid, just like if you spill cow milk, so you'll need to wash them routinely. If you have two, and one is in the wash, you'll have a second ready to go. Having a pumping bra will allow you to multitask like the queen you are and help keep the stiffness out of your neck and lower back muscles.

Would you rather stoop over a pump and hold the milk bottles while they slowly fill, or have your bra do the job for you? Get two.

Want two big ticket items to prioritize for your house? Here's what you need to protect your white gold:

Deep Freezer

You can freeze breast milk. You want to freeze breast milk. You want to stockpile as much as you can, especially if you will return to work or be away from your baby before their first birthday. You always start with the oldest milk, then work your way forward. Get a deep freezer with an auto defrost.

So, what's the second house item we needed and worried over because we didn't have it?

A generator.

Gas Powered Generator

Our biggest fear was that our power would go out during a hurricane or after a storm, and the milk I worked so hard for would go to waste. T.J. and I both lost sleep over the possibility of losing our white gold harvest. We bought a gas-powered generator when I was pregnant. Over the course of nursing and pumping for each kid, it did actually save our butts several times when we lost power.

Pro Tip: A Wireless Temperature Monitor is a great accessory to add. Have you ever accidently not closed the fridge or freezer all the way, and found it hours later with warm food or drinks inside? Me too. Grab a monitor if your freezer will be in a basement, garage, or out of the way so you don't lose sleep too!

Getting married, moving, or having a baby in a short time frame? Call the generator or freezer a wedding or housewarming present, especially if this is not your first baby and others think "you have all the gear you need". Go for house stuff!

THE BEST DEAL IN TOWN

OK, great. I just added literally thousands of dollars of gear to your baby prep list. Where can you pinch your pennies to afford all the other things you need? If the price tag on the must-have gear is too much, seriously look into pre-loved merch.

I plan my weekends around consignment sales, AKA The Best Deal in Town. I wish I'd known about these sales sooner!! It's like a yard sale on steroids. It's like Supermarket Sweep for moms on a budget.

If you live near any large cities, there should be one or several options for these sales. They are not created equal!

Some are for profit, so the items are more expensive. There are also non-profit clubs or groups that host these as their major fundraisers and use the consignor fee income to pay for their support system and social networking. My favorite sale is put on by our local Mothers of Multiples group.

If you don't have access to a local sale, or the timing doesn't work out for you, don't stress. My friends find great deals on Craigslist, Nextdoor, OfferUp, and Facebook Marketplace.

What are the best grabs?
Back-up nursing pillows and covers for when the one with the spit up is in the wash. Pack and Plays, baby clothes, maternity clothes, and ergo carriers. You will pay pennies on the dollar for these!

Does used gear ick you out? Me too. I sanitize used soft items that fit in the dryer. For the clothes and nursing pillows, I dry them first, on high heat, for ten minutes. Then I wash them as if they were new.

For large Pack and Plays, baby tubs, and other hard items, you can use a bleach solution or your favorite germ-killing wipes to clean them; then let them air dry.

Reminder to be careful with recalls, especially for cribs, bassinets, and car seats. Research the latest guidelines or check online for the specific item and "born on" date.

Go with a friend! Ask people you know with kids where they get deals on kids' gear. If one of them says it's a consignment sale, find out about how to score a VIP pass. To raise more money, many of these sales have

VIP passes you can buy. They reserve opening night hours for pass holders.

Spend a couple bucks on the pass, so you get first dibs for quality and pricing. The larger sales could have two dozen Pack and Plays—and usually a few duplicate items. You want the cheapest, nicest one, right? The pass is worth it!

Chapter 9 Key Points
- Use your baby registry for the best support gear.
- Don't spend big bucks on baby furniture.
- Having a baby is the best excuse to invest in a deep freezer and generator.
- Consignment sales are life.
- Do ten Kegels right now.

CHAPTER TEN

MEDICAL AND NATURAL TREATMENTS YOU CAN START IN THE SECOND TRIMESTER

K-taping and foam rolling have become trendy online, in clinics, and at home. Here's how you can be your own trendsetter along with my Pro Tips for success!

FOAM ROLLING/SELF MASSAGE

In the biz we call this "Instrument Assisted Soft Tissue Mobilization" (IASTM).

This is when you use a tool to break up knots or thick spots in your muscles and soft tissues.

Expect any item to sell for a higher price if it carries labels like "baby", "wedding", or "fitness". To save some money, I'll show you what you can use from around your house instead.

For Your Back
Pro Tip: Use these day-to-day lower budget items to work out your own kinks after a bad day.

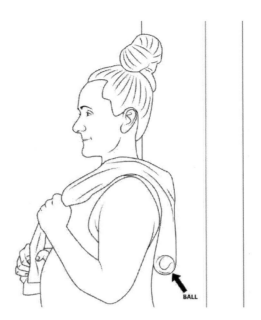

o **Self Massage with a tennis or lacrosse ball.**
- Use what you've already got.
- Place the ball between you and the wall and slowly move your body up and down and side to side to massage your sore back or shoulder muscles.
- If you like the pressure hard, a lacrosse ball will do the trick, as it's denser. If you cringe with too-hard pressure, a tennis ball is more your speed.
- Put a sock on it! If you have trouble reaching to place the ball between you and the wall, put the ball in a long sock, and lower it into place.

For Your Hips and Calves

○ **Foam Roller.**

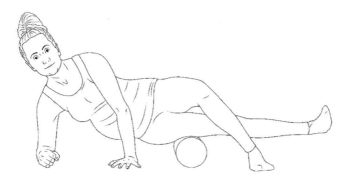

- ▪ **Hips:** Place the foam roller (12 or 36 inch, full-foam roller) between you and the wall, or between you and the floor. Roll it back and forth on the outside of your hips.

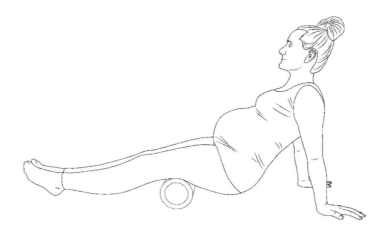

- ▪ **Back of your legs:** Sit on the floor with your legs stretched out in front of you. You can do both legs at the same time, or one at a time. Use your arms to control your body, and rock forward and back. The roller goes under your thighs if your hamstrings are sore or tight, or under your calves if they are sore or tight.

- Foam Rollers come in variable hardness. Typically, the 'soft' or 'standard' foam rollers are tolerated better because you can lean more of your weight into it, or hold it on your sore spot a little longer to get deeper. 'Extra firm' rollers are also available if you prefer the deeper pressure.

For Your Shoulder Blades
- o **TheraCane.**
  - This thing is awesome! If you have someone at home who will rub your shoulders every single time you ask, you won't need one of these. But if you're like me and need a hand (or have someone willing to rub you but who presses a little too hard) this is a game-changer.
  - The first year we were in physical therapy school, our class ordered TheraCanes in bulk for ourselves and to give as gifts. My TheraCane gets heavy use and is holding up after over 15 years.
  - It's like a shepherd's crook. You hold the handle and the knobs on the ends massage between your shoulder blades. It's also one of the only ways you can really massage your own upper trapezius, the muscle that connects your neck to the top of your shoulders and often holds a lot of tension.

For Headaches
- o **Occipital Release Tool.**
  - This is like a cradle for your head. You use its finger-shaped ridges to self-massage the back of your head, and you control the pressure. If you have a computer or desk job or you're spending too much time on your phone researching your latest "getting ready for baby" obsession (or after the

baby comes and you're spending hours looking into their perfect little face), you'll love this.

- Phase 1: Lie on your back with your knees bent. Place the Occipital Release Tool under the base of your skull, and gently scoot your body toward the foot of the bed. Relax. Let the muscles in the back of your neck soften up as you relax. You can stay here for a few minutes.

- Phase 2: Add movement. Try turning your head slowly from right to left. Try nodding your head gently. Do five to ten times each.

- Want a lower-budget option? Take a long sock and place two tennis balls inside. Tie a knot to keep the balls snugly in place. Works nearly the same, and it's cheaper.

- Don't forget your posture! Do you get pretty bad tension headaches that worsen as the week goes on but disappear on the weekends? Look at your workstation and work posture.

KINESIOLOGY TAPING

AKA Kinesio Taping AKA K-taping.

You may have seen people walking (or running) around town with strips of tape located on their arms and legs. If so, you're familiar with K-tape.

K-tape is a latex-free, medical-grade tape made of cotton and elastic. The sticky part of the tape is activated by your body heat. It stays on for one to three days, even if it gets wet in the shower.

Why use K-tape? For lift and support. To relieve pressure and ease pain due to joint and muscle soreness in your back, shoulders, feet, or your sorest muscle.[36] And it's also safe on your baby-belly. I'll even share a technique that helps with swollen, sore ankles. If you're pregnant and it's warm outside (or in!), tape can make you less sweaty than a brace.

People often find it provides better "fits me like a glove" support than a brace, and tape has a great short-term effect on pain relief. You should see an immediate change after putting it on. Exercise or get moving after you put the tape on to remind your body how to move with less pain.

Who can use it? It's not just for pro athletes! K-tape popularity grew big-time after people started seeing it on professional athletes and Olympic volleyball players and swimmers on TV, but anybody can use it. With a little practice, you'll be a pro before you get to the end of your first roll of tape.

When can't I use it? Don't ever tape over irritated skin or an open wound. Even though it is latex-free, if you are sensitive to the adhesive of some bandages or you're "allergic to everything," monitor your skin closely. If it feels itchy, red, or hot under the tape, carefully remove it. Also, if the tape makes your pain worse or flares up a new pain, take the tape off right away.

Make sure your skin is free of lotion before taping. Use rubbing alcohol to gently clean your skin before taping.

Pro Tip: When you are gathering your gear, add one more thing to your cart. Milk of Magnesia. It's #1 use is obviously to coat your stomach and protect it from acid irritation, but guess what? If you take a washcloth or paper towel and apply a light smear to your skin after it's clean, it will protect you from skin irritation *and* make the tape stick better!

Where do I get started? Try these at home, but if you run into trouble, have a professional (like a physical therapist experienced with taping) put the tape on you the first time. After you learn the ins and outs, it's a great thing to continue to do on yourself, or have your partner help you with. You can buy the tape at many drug stores or from the physical therapy clinic.

Which brand is the best? For pregnancy, Rock Tape is extra sticky and good to use with exercise or if you sweat easily. Kinesio Tex Gold is nice if you have more sensitive skin.

This is the most technical chapter in the book, but I want to give you all the natural options possible to get you through pain.

There's an instruction paper in the box of tape on how to achieve 25% and 50% tension. If you lay the tape down gently as you peel the paper backing off, that is 25%. Gently pulling while you lay the tape down is 50%. If you pull both ends of the tape until it cannot stretch anymore, that is 100% tension.

How do I use it? Now that you've gotten a crash course in using tape, here's the moment you've been waiting for: the best places to put this colorful tape!

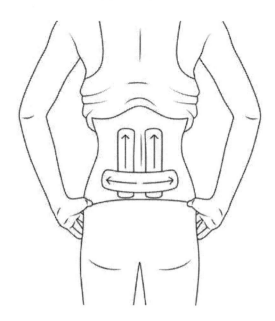

- ○ **Lower Back H Technique**
  Most popular for back pain: This helps back pain and muscle spasms and is easy for someone to put on for you. It's also a reminder for good posture.
    - ▪ Cut three strips.
    - ▪ Stand up and bend forward to put the tape on.
    - ▪ Strips 1 and 2 each start at the dimple in your lower back, and you pull them up toward your bra strap with 25% tension. On strip three, use 50% tension and lay it horizontally over the area of pain in your lower back.

Pro Tip: Do not pull on ends of the tape. Lay them down gently without any pull. If the ends have tension, you might see your skin red and irritated when you take the tape off. You'll need to take a few days off from taping and let your skin breathe.

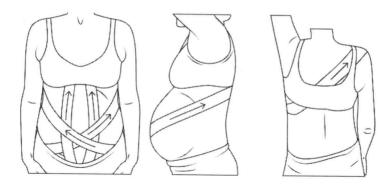

o **The Belly Sling**

Baby bump weighing you down or hurting your back? Here's a custom support sling that supports from your bump to your back.

- Cut two strips that are each about three feet long to start. You can add two extra strips in the front if the first two didn't provide enough relief.

- Stand up. Place the end of the first piece at the front of the hip. Raise the opposite arm. Apply the tape in a spiral pattern, pulling toward the raised arm with 50% tension, under the belly and around to the opposite shoulder blade. It will tuck a few inches under your bra strap. Repeat this on the other side.

- Extra Lift Strips: Cut two more strips, 15 inches long each. Raise your arms up. Start one piece of tape on the front of your pelvic bone and pull up with 50% tension over your stomach to the ribcage. The tape will stop under your bra again. Repeat on the other side. These two strips should be like the lanes on a road, with your belly button in the middle of the road.

Pro Tip: Use scissors to round the edges of each piece of tape, so your clothes pull on it less and it stays in place better, for longer.

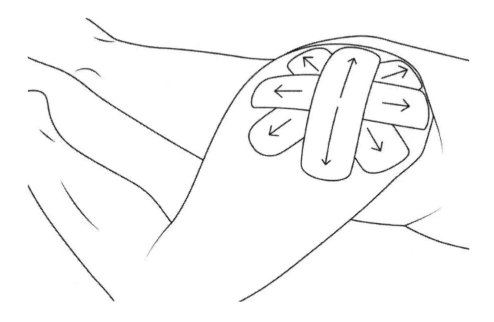

o **X Marks the Spot**

Can you put your hand on a super sore knot on your hips or butt and say it hurts "right here"? Or is your foot falling asleep, as it might when you sit on it strangely? If so, then this is the technique for you.

- Lie on your side with your top leg rolled forward to gently stretch your butt.

- Cut two to four strips, each six to eight inches long. Remove the middle third of the paper backing from each strip. Pull with 50% tension and place the exposed part of the tape directly over your sore spot or on your butt where the sciatic nerve is being pressured. Remove the paper for each end, and lay down the tape without tension. Repeat this with the remaining strips.

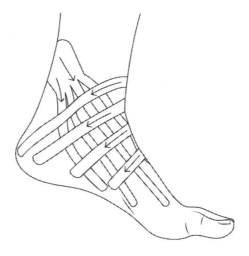

o **Swollen Feet**

My swelling was the worst in the last two months of both of my pregnancies. Are your "dogs barking", or do you feel like your toes are little sausages now? Try this tape technique.

- Sit down with your leg straight out in front of you on a chair or the bed. Flex your toes toward your face.
- Cut two strips, six to eight inches long each. Now for the arts and crafts! Hold one end of the strip and cut a slit longways, leaving 2 inches uncut. The tape looks like a Y.
- Cut each part of your Y further into thin strips. Now you have your two-inch handle and a fan with four little tails. Do this to your second strip.
- Anchor the handle at your mid-shin, and gently lay the tape down with 25% tension, softly pressing each tail down toward your foot, making the 4 tails look like a folding hand fan. Take the handle from strip #2 and turn it 90° from your first piece. Now lay the four tails down with 25% tension toward your foot. If you're feeling extra fancy, use two different tape colors.

111

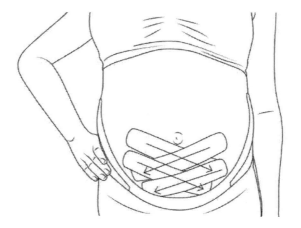

o **Diastasis Recti**

Depending on how tan your skin is, you may have a darker line right down the middle of your abs. Use that as your midline for this technique. If you're super pale like me, draw an imaginary line downward from your breastbone toward your belly button.

- While standing, gently contract your ab muscles (this is optional. Do this the second time you try this technique. Some find that this makes the tape feel too tight).

- Apply one end of the strip just under the lowest rib you can feel. No tension. Pull down at a diagonal toward your pubic bone using 75% pull. Place the other side of the X starting from the top, then pull down using 75% stretch. 75% will feel tight, but this will loosen up as you wear it.

- X #2- should overlap the first X by one-half to one cm. Repeat the overlapping tapes until the area of separation is covered. This may end just above your pubic hair. The number of Xs you need depends on how long the split portion of your abs is. Typically, three to four Xs will do the trick.

This is one you can do yourself in front of a mirror, or have your partner apply as with the other techniques.

Pro Tip: Ready to take the tape off? Get it nice and soapy during the second shower you take after it's been on, and gently peel it off. Three days on and one day off will keep your skin healthy.

Phew! You made it.

DRY NEEDLING

If K-tape was the first on-trend natural-healing technique you've seen all over social media, then dry needling is probably the second. The cool thing is both are pretty affordable things you can look to if your back pain is holding you back!

Dry needling is a technique used to treat pain that comes from your muscles. A small, solid needle is placed directly into the muscle knot or spot that hurts to help break the pain cycle.

Dry needling eliminates pain, knots, and tension, and improves how you move without medication by:
  o Stopping chemicals your body releases that trigger pain.
  o Relieving stubborn muscle knots.
  o Helping your body move better once the muscle knots are gone.
  o Allowing you to use your muscles the right way when they don't hurt.

Who does it help?
  o Anyone with neck, back, shoulder, or arm pain.
  o Someone who experiences headaches, even headaches caused by jaw pain, migraines, or tension.
  o Someone with leg pain or pain in the butt (sciatica, hamstring strains, calf tightness or spasm).

How is dry needling different from acupuncture? Both use thin needles, but dry needling uses typically one at a time, where acupuncture uses many. Acupuncture typically leaves the needles in for an extended period of time in the skin. For dry needling, they are placed directly into the muscle knot for a minute or so each.

Does it hurt? Most people say they don't even feel the needle go in. When the muscle reacts to the needle many feel a deep cramping sensation, which is a good result. The relief or benefits are felt later once the muscle knot is gone.

How many treatments does it typically take? Typically, it takes several visits to get a positive reaction to take place. We are trying to get the body to ease the knots, get the body to stop releasing the pain chemicals, and allow your body to finally move normally. One session may reduce the pain and shrink the area that hurts, but each additional application helps reduce pain and get you back to normal, faster.

I put dry needling in a second trimester chapter for a reason. There are so many changes going on in your body during trimester one that I wouldn't recommend this. Cautious therapists will ask you to wait until the second trimester, before you can do the dry needling. It is mildly invasive, since the thin needle goes into your muscle.

There are some spots that are no-fly zones when you're pregnant, but I've seen some amazing things with dry needling later in pregnancy. Avoid anywhere on your trunk that would be too close to your uterus, such as your abdomen, lumbar spine, and sacrum.

I had a first-time mom that suffered through her second trimester before we met her for PT. She had been a regular at the gym. She'd tried several things to relieve her pain, and while a few helped her pain a little, nothing knocked it out. Her back hurt so badly she couldn't walk or go to the gym.

She begged me to dry needle the muscles in her butt. It really was amazing! We did needling for three sessions, once a week, and she got back to the gym. She hadn't worked out in months, but thanks to the dry needling, her last weeks prior to her baby's arrival were pain free. I really saw those tiny needles work their magic.

I called her three weeks after the baby arrived to check in. She was so happy that her back pain stayed gone after her dry needling success. She was still feeling good, postpartum. And most importantly, she and the baby were doing great.

DIET

"Ugh. Diet."
Yes, diet!

How much weight did your OBGYN tell you to gain for the entire time you're pregnant? Mine told me 35 pounds. I was like *yessssss*. I'm eating for two. I can't wait!

Woo hoo! A doctor told me to eat more. After counting calories, painfully watching TV shows about delicious food while my more-healthy food digested in my tummy to "maintain a healthy weight" to start with the best pre-baby body I could, this was a challenge I was *happy* to accept.

We can't talk about natural healing options for your pregnant body without talking about food. You are what you eat. If you put garbage in, you'll feel like garbage. If you eat better, avoid fried food, and eat more fruits and veggies, you really will feel better too.

Easy, right?

Not so fast. Things that can go wrong:

Eating All The Food

I raced to the finish line with my second pregnancy. I gained over 20 pounds *fast*. Watch out for stretch marks!

Glucose Tests

At 24 to 28 weeks, your doctor will give you a lab slip and tell you to schedule a resting glucose test. This checks to see how your body is responding to the pregnancy, specifically screening for gestational diabetes.

You go to the lab in the morning with an empty stomach and drink a sugar drink. Then you wait an hour and have your blood drawn. Days later you'll find out the results.

For Baby #1 I was right on track, no problems. I took my resting glucose test and was pleasantly surprised that the sugar drink they gave me was like a slightly thickened, orange sports drink. All my mom friends warned me about how nasty it was. Maybe since I expected the worst, it was no big deal.

Baby #2 was a different story. I took my resting glucose test and failed it. The nurse at the doctor's office said the numbers were pretty bad. What?! I was a rule follower, especially with anything that kept the baby healthy.

I was super bummed. It's not unusual to feel devastated, ashamed, or have several days where you feel depressed after news like this.

I thought the "eating for two" label would justify my sweet tooth. The failed glucose test happened directly following my birthday and Halloween, which are just 10 days apart. I did not hold back. I was eating for two, after all, and these are two of my favorite days of the year!

When you fail your one-hour resting glucose test, you go back a few weeks later to take a three-hour test. I was tired and fasting (AKA "hangry") but tried to keep myself busy while I waited.

During pregnancy, hormones that help your baby grow also reduce how well your insulin works, thus allowing your blood sugar to rise. Other factors that make healthy blood sugar an uphill climb are being over the age of 30, having a Body Mass Index (BMI) over 25, or having a close blood-relative who has Diabetes. Interestingly, I passed the test at the age of 29, but I failed at the age of 31.

Limiting extra sugar in your blood during pregnancy is important to protect your and the baby's health and development. If one of your tests comes back abnormal, your doctor will suggest some changes. Diet and exercise are the two factors that you have the most control over. If there's room for improvement in either, making changes here can have the most impact on your bloodwork.

For me, I needed to make the most changes with the sweets in my diet. After a few changes, I did pass the three-hour test. I recommend taking the one-hour test somewhat seriously. I passed the second test because I stopped chugging orange juice and cut way back on my "eating for two" servings of candy and dessert.

The test measures how much sugar is running around in your blood. Eating less sugar leading up to the test means better results.

Failed glucose tests happen every day. Everyone has different background factors to keep in mind. Tackle your diet and exercise head on to avoid any complications with your pregnancy. Know that you should not be ashamed when you are working hard in the diet and exercise department.

See Chapter 13 for how to find a nutritionist if you need a little more help with this.

Partner Sympathy Weight Gain

Yes, this is a real thing. If you or your partner buy two (or four!) cartons of ice cream every week, you're not the only one gaining weight this season. Expecting-partner weight gain is real. It's part of most of our journeys.

Is there any hope? Yes. Make plans to take walks or hikes together. If you already have one child in a stroller, this may feel impossible to schedule around work, naps, and life in general. Sit down and schedule two walks per week. Walks for our family take time to finesse, but during the weeks we prioritize family walks, everyone gets along better, too.

Avoid excess weight gain for you both. Embrace your accountability buddies: your partner, your mom, best friend, or neighbor.

Chapter 10 Key Points
- Kinesiology taping is for pregnant ladies, too.
- Learn self-massage.
- Dry needling can break up tension in a muscle knot if the massage didn't work.
- Watch your sugar intake when you're eating for two.
- Do ten Kegels right now.

CHAPTER ELEVEN

PRODUCTS YOU NEED IN THE THIRD TRIMESTER

Happy 27th Week! You've entered the Nesting Phase! You're getting close to meeting your bambino/bambina! To me, this was a huge relief.

So, what other gear could you possibly need that we haven't already covered?

COMPRESSION SOCKS

Knee-high socks with compression. Oh, so sexy.

The weight of your baby is sitting on the veins in the top of your legs. This makes it hard for the fluid in your ankles to fight gravity and circulate around your body. The fluid gets stuck in your legs, making them feel swollen and heavy. If you ignore it, long-time pressure can be a factor for varicose or "spider" veins in your legs in the future. *Super* sexy.

Compression socks help with circulation, reduce pain, and can prevent those varicose veins. During the last six-eight weeks, the socks were a *must* for me, but you can start wearing these bad boys any time in the third trimester, or sooner if you need to.

Wear them during the day when you're on your feet more, and let your legs breathe when you're sleeping at night. In bed, the gravity factor is neutralized, and your legs don't need the help of the compression as much.

You do not need the hospital variety that go all the way up to your hips. Find a pair of knee highs that fit your normal shoe size and offer light to medium compression, in the ballpark of 8-20mm/Hg. "Mm/Hg" is a unit of pressure; basically, the higher the number, the tighter the socks.

Start with two pairs. If you like them, get enough to last your laundry week! They have nude and black socks if you need that for work, but compression socks come in every fun pattern you can image!

HIP-SHAPING BELT

This is something you'll need after you deliver the baby, but buy it *now* because you only have a six- to eight-week window of time to get your hips to return to your pre-baby slimness.

Many complain that their curves change, like their hips get wider after having kids. The relaxin in your body can cause long-lasting effects, and many women do have wider hips after having kids. I'm not talking about the post baby fluff that takes some time to get off. The actual measurements of the width of your hips expands during pregnancy to allow for birth.

If you liked your pre-baby hips or worry about after-baby back pain due to loose ligaments, getting a hip-shaping belt can get your hips back in shape. It looks like several other lower back stability belts, but a hip-shaping belt can be the key to regaining that pre-baby figure.

The hip-shaping belt helps the ligaments stabilize back to their pre-pregnancy place. If you have back pain during any pregnancy, or you've ever battled with constant or off-and-on back pain before you even got pregnant, having a "loosey-goosey" back is going to wreck the stability of that area.

I totally missed out on this after #1. That's part of why my back hurt so much when I was pregnant with #2.

Don't make the same mistake I did.

Future you will be like, "Thanks, Past Me, you are so smart!"

Chapter 11 Key Points
- o   Feel light on your feet by wearing compression socks.
- o   A hip shaping belt helps get your pre-baby body back.
- o   Do ten Kegels right now.

CHAPTER TWELVE

THIRD TRIMESTER PLANNING AND DELIVERY

How do you prepare for the physical and emotional aspects of giving birth? Plan ahead while you still can, before you get "all the emotions".

CLASSES

I didn't grow up helping with babies. I have one brother, and we're exactly two years apart—we have the same birthday! No diapers to change there. All my younger cousins live in other states. I didn't do much babysitting. I'd never even changed a single diaper before I had my first child.

Because of this, I dragged T.J. to a couple of prenatal classes. He was eight when his brother was born, and had diaper changing experience. He just needed to learn the differences for diapering girls.

If you lack time spent with babies, you should check out a class or two. If you feel like a pro, and elect to skip the classes, here are the biggest things I learned in the ones we took.

Nursing and Lactation Consultants

If you plan to nurse, find a lactation consultant. The hospital where we delivered had a full-timer that came to see you while you were there. She was amazing.

We got her email address, and we used it! We still send her pictures of the girls after a healthy check-up with their doctor.

I hit a few walls during breastfeeding, and she helped me overcome them. Find yourself a resource for when you hit a wall with breastfeeding.

Happiest Baby on The Block

This resource was referenced during our baby care class. Simple, mind blowing stuff. Check my references at the end of the book for the full details.[37] There is a DVD and a book. Get one of those.

Swaddling is a game-changer. Learn how to use an old-fashioned swaddle, but also get a set of these modern swaddles. After a few short weeks, our babies "Houdinied" out of my best "burrito baby", old-fashioned swaddle job.

It's so fun to free a little baby from a swaddle. Freshly un-swaddled babies have the *best,* cutest stretches *ever!* Our swaddled babies slept better. Get your swaddle on.

BABY HOLDING PREP

My purpose in writing this book is to teach you how to feel better in your back, body, and mind while you're pregnant. But while we're here in your pregnant mind, let's get mentally and physically ready to carry this baby around after they arrive, and *not* get new muscles sore when that happens.

Typically, new moms have huge knots in their upper traps, the muscle that connects your shoulders to your neck. By doing your rows and bicep curls from Chapter 5, you'll train your muscles for your up and coming new job!

It could be reaching down for a laundry basket, a paperclip from the floor, or even getting jugs of juice or milk out of the fridge. Start lifting and carrying day-to-day things like this:[38]

How to Lift

- Kneel down beside the object you need to pick up.
- Bring the item close to you.
- Use your free hand to help you push your body up to a half kneel. One foot steps forward, while the knee and foot of the back leg are still on the floor.
- Stand up, hugging your baby or the item close to your chest or stomach.
- Always carry your child (or object) by hugging it close to your body.
- When it's a baby you're picking up, press your hand against their stomach. A baby will flex and bend their hips, thus making it easier to lift them.

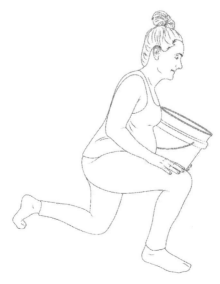

Lifting from floor posture

Get Your Baby-Holding Muscles Pumped Up

You've got a good foundation. All the Kegels you're doing are keeping your pelvic muscles in condition. You know how to turn your abs on. (If you've gotten too busy to keep up with your exercises, jump back to Chapter 5 for the strengthening exercises.)

Now, let's flex those Mommy Guns. Pump up your baby-carrying muscles and get your body ready for lots of holding, and snuggles!

FOOD STOCK

Buy Double

When I was pregnant, I got in the habit of buying twice as many of the items on my list as I needed. If you have the resources to stock up, do it! Why make another trip for the same refried beans that you like for the next Taco Tuesday? Just get double now.

Pro Tip: Stock up on things that your partner enjoys making.

Freeze A Duplicate

I'm inspired by (and big-time envious of) anyone that posts online about all the food they cook ahead in order to have home-cooking waiting for them after work. I've never figured this one out on a large scale—and not all of our faves freeze well.

During the third trimester of my second pregnancy, I did make this one epic change: once a week I made something that *did* freeze well. For me it was lasagna, an enchilada casserole, and another casserole we made all the time. Instead of making just the one we would eat that night, I made a second and froze it in an aluminum pan, covered with plastic wrap and aluminum foil.

I at least had a few choices for "home cooking waiting for us" on days we were absolutely too pooped to cook.

Grocery Delivery

For me, this would go in the next chapter: Not Your First Rodeo, because I didn't discover this life-bettering service until I had two in diapers.

Especially if I had to juggle more than one kid, I never did figure out how to fit all the groceries around the carrier if kid one was in the front, and if kid two doesn't have head support yet. The two-seater carts won't work.

What store do you buy most of your groceries from? If they have their own website and service in place, use them. If they do not, check to see if they work with Instacart. Instacart has shoppers that can do your shopping at various stores that don't have their own service.

My grocery store was so easy to work with. All the things I'd bought in previous months (all logged when they scanned my loyalty card) pulled forward onto a checklist. This made it easy to buy again and add any new items. You do have to plan a little bit in advance, so have your shopping order ready and entered two days (varies by service) before you need your stuff.

A MALPOSITIONED BABY

Back Labor: Myth or Fact?

Fact. Back labor is when the back of your baby's head presses on your spine and tailbone during labor. It's not fun. I had it with both of mine. Here's some tips to try to get that baby to face the right way.

The human skull is made up of 22 separate bones. Many of these have fissure lines, kind of like the tectonic plates in the earth, where different plates meet. An infant's skull bones have not fully turned to bone by the time they're born. This gives their soft skull more give so it can pass through your birth canal with more ease. Phew!

If your baby is head down, with their adorable little smooched face pointing toward your butt, the two soft spots they have are in good position, and the diameter of their head is at a better angle to pass through the birth canal. It feels smaller due to this angle.

However, some babies end up with their face looking at your belly button.

When your baby is head down, but facing forward, you can say they are "sunny-side up", or a "star-gazer". The medical jargon for this is "occiput posterior". You can get a gander at this on ultrasound. Your baby bump may also feel softer, or you might feel baby kicking around the middle of your belly instead of kicking your ribs.

The back pain you feel during back labor is intense, and different than the aches you feel during pregnancy. The good news is that even in the cramped quarters of nine months pregnant, the baby can still get into the right position! Here's the exercise you need to reduce the chance of back labor:

Rocking on Hands and Knees
Get on the floor on your hands and knees, or put your arms on an ottoman or the seat cushion of a couch. Rock front to back, rock your butt side to side, rock your hips in circles, first clockwise, then counterclockwise.

The best time to do this is after you eat. The calories really get the baby active, and you have a better chance of getting their little body to roll and face the right way. Do this for five minutes per day, after one or every meal.

The baby will continue to move into and out of the correct-facing way. If you show up for go-time and the baby is still sunny side up, your doctor may be able to help get the baby into the right position.

Both of my babies were sunny-side up when their deliveries started, despite this being one of my go-to third trimester exercises. I would feel their arms and legs push and kick me in different places, so it did feel like they were in the right spot sometimes and facing the wrong direction other times.

During contractions my OB, Dr. P, would put his hands on the baby (inside me, while the baby was still inside) and try to get her to turn 180 degrees. Guess what? It worked the first time. Hallelujah! That baby weighed in at 8lb, 2oz.

Guess what else?! It didn't work the second time. Baby #2 weighed 8lb, 9 oz and her shoulders must have been that much broader. She almost got stuck. It hurt. *A lot.* But Dr. P helped me push her out anyway, and she and I both made it through healthy!

I had a room full of people ready to whisk me into emergency surgery if my last attempt at pushing didn't work. I was super surprised when a dozen people cheered when #2 came out on my last push.

After we made it through the labor, Dr. P actually told my husband, "I'm not delivering any more of your children. No more babies. At least give me a couple years off." We laughed.

Breech Baby

A breech baby is when, by the last four weeks of pregnancy, the baby is feet down instead of head down. About 3-5% of pregnancies have this issue. Some doctors may recommend medication, or an intervention to try to avoid a C-section, however evidence is not very clear on success rates of all the options.[39] This is another area to "talk to your doctor" about your options.

BIRTH PLAN

This is definitely something my mom didn't sit down and type up. A birth plan is a document that outlines your labor and delivery preferences. It includes things like: Birthing center vs hospital, pushing the baby out vs C-section, is Tramadol or an epidural OK, and how many nights are you planning to stay at the hospital after delivery?

It puts all your wishes in one place for your healthcare team to review.[40] They're called delivery "preferences", as these things are your Plan A. Birth plans oftentimes change in the moment. Regardless, if you put your plan on paper, your medical team will consider these preferences and have back-up plans as needed to keep you and the baby safe.

I actually took a 55cm diameter Swiss Ball in with me to the hospital to deliver my first baby. Being the smarty-pants mom-to-be who worked in health care, I knew best! Sitting on the ball and bouncing was going to ease the pain of my contractions and put my baby in the right place, so my labor would be easy-peasy.

The check-in nurse on the labor and delivery floor of the hospital straight-up laughed at me. Like, "OK Mama, you do you, but you're not going to be needing that silly ball." She was right.

I got sent home because I wasn't dilated at all, and labor was going super-slow. After waiting for hours and hours and feeling like labor must have progressed enough to admit me for The Big Show, T.J. and I went back to the hospital. I left the ball at home.

Put what fits your ideal birth-day on the plan. Or don't write up a plan. Either way, your team will ask you the important questions and do what they need to do to get the baby here as safely as possible.

So often the reality of our situation doesn't match our best laid plans. Especially for first time moms. There's a good chance your birth plan isn't going to shake out perfectly. Don't let yourself, or others, put too much pressure on following the map you've laid out.

Some moms who plan a natural route end up needing a C-section. Having a C-section is not a fail, to yourself or your baby. If your immediate situation necessitates a shift, your birth plan will flow to the new options. Birth plans are meant to be fluid documents.

Besides the medical plan, what about the rest of your life? What arrangements do you make when you travel, or don't sleep in your own bed? Have a talk with your babysitter and/or pet sitter to discuss what you need for help, and if they'll be available to help when the time comes.

DELIVERY DAY

Here you are. You made it. It. Is. Go. Time. Birth plan in hand, hospital bag packed. Or not. Babies come when they're ready!

My very thorough doctor warned me up front that my babies could be too big for me to push out if they went full term. I'm 5'2". T.J. is a 6'5" Viking.

My eyes glazed over and I said, "Gotcha."

He said, "No, really. That's one reason C-sections happen; the baby physically cannot come out. You could have a problem." He strongly endorsed delivering in a hospital, in case my Plan A to push them out didn't work. The medical team to perform a C-section would be in-house, if needed.

I said, "Sounds great!"

So, both of my beautiful babies were delivered at the hospital. Strangely enough, at the same hospital where I was born!

Perineal Massage

A perineal massage is where your doctor or someone certified in prenatal massage actually stretches the tissues surrounding your birth canal. It helps cut down on the chance you'll tear or need an episiotomy (a surgical cut made at the opening of the vagina) when you give birth.[41]

Does this actually work? Heck yea. My doctor did this during my labor with both girls. He basically used his hands to pre-stretch things during several of my contractions.

It helped so, so much to keep things flexible "down there". Put it on your list to ask about.

Frog Leg Assistants

I pushed from a standard position: lying on your back, head inclined, knees bent, legs out like a frog. T.J. held one leg. A nurse held the other. They were a huge mismatch! If your partner is ready for a front row-seat for this, chat with them about matching the pressure of your other leg-holder. If there is a mismatch, it's easier for your pubic bones to get out of whack.

The good news is, a good PT can line you back up after your "6-8 weeks post-delivery" visit if your pubic bone is painful or popping. Just a little tip to avoid that issue, if possible.

Get Up and Move After

If you say "yes" to an epidural, or even if you don't use one, wait until your medical team OKs you to get up and out of bed. An epidural numbs the intense pain of contractions so you can't feel that pain, but that means you can't feel your legs either. Your legs will literally feel ten times as heavy and won't be strong enough for you to stand.

After the epidural medicine wears off enough, and you've received the OK, use someone by your side if needed, and *do* get up. Get up as often as your doctor says to. Lying in bed too much can cause blood to pool in your torn-up and trying-to-heal uterus, or in your legs.

Get up routinely to keep your blood circulating in your legs and uterus. This will help prevent any blood clots following delivery.

Chapter 12 Key Points

- o Find out if your hospital or birthing center has a lactation consultant. Say hello!
- o Practice your swaddling.
- o Do your rows and bicep curls three times this week, if you weren't already.
- o Always carry babies and heavy things by hugging them close to your body.
- o Stock up the food in your pantry and freezer.

o Write up a birth plan, but don't be surprised if you don't use it or if it changes.

o Ask your OB if they do a perineal massage during labor.

o Do ten Kegels right now.

CHAPTER THIRTEEN

WHEN DO I ASK FOR HELP?

YOU ARE NOT ALONE

"It takes a village to raise a child." ~African proverb

Really! Family. Friends. Your extended medical people. Online groups. In-person groups. All of these will say, "I've got your back." You just have to let them.

DAY TO DAY TASKS

Are you gasping for breath by the time you go up one flight of stairs? Is it even worse when you're carrying something, even if you didn't think it was that heavy? This is normal. Take one step at a time if you need to catch your breath.

If doing stairs hurts your back or knees, this would be a great time to ask for help schlepping things up the stairs, bending down to reach low things, or even tying your shoes. You're growing a human inside of you and making your own sacrifices these months. Ask for some help.

PHYSICAL THERAPY

Ask for help sooner rather than later. Put the discomfort behind you and experience the joy you are meant to! Visit a therapist as soon as your pains don't go away after using my tips for 48 hours. Oftentimes, a tight or weak muscle can throw off the balance of your back, shoulder, etc.

Revisit Chapter 6 for "How to Find a Good PT" if it's time to make a call.

Pelvic Health and Pelvic Floor Dysfunction

What is this? If you Google any of the keywords here, it's a crapshoot what info will turn up. Basically, there are several layers of muscles and connective tissues that make up the floor under your bladder, uterus and rectum. If the muscles are tight or weak, you can have problems.

There are four categories that pelvic floor function could fall into: normal, underactive, overactive (tight or pain), or non-functioning (often both weak and painful).[42]

What does pelvic floor dysfunction feel like? Pressure or pain during or after sex or going to the bathroom. Also issues with incontinence, which may include excessive leaking or incomplete bladder emptying. This often causes you to go again after you just went. These are things a pelvic floor PT can help you with.

What exactly does treatment look like? How hands-on are we talking here? Treatments take the same amount of time or are sometimes longer than a typical PT appointment for something muscle or joint related, such as back pain.

Like muscles in every other part of your body, if they are tight, weak, or have coordination issues, exercises and re-teaching the muscles how to do their jobs better will help. Is the word "Kegel" starting to sound familiar?

There are hands-on techniques too. If you have any scar tissue or stubborn muscle knots, a PT that specializes in Pelvic Health can also put on gloves and perform an internal vaginal or rectal treatment to address your problem area. These treatments are always performed in a private treatment room after you talk with the therapist.

They'll explain your treatment choices, and you'll agree to the option that meets your needs. At this point, if the pain is spoiling the intimacy you have in your life, or you're tired of being in Tinkle Town, why not?

What kind of extra certifications would a PT need to perform internal vaginal releases? We don't get enough experience with this in school. Additional mentoring is needed in this area after completing physical therapy school.

PTs can get a Women's Health Specialist Certification. However, the specialist certification did not come about until 2009. There are many PTs without the certification who have years of experience. To find an experienced therapist in your area, search the 'Academy of Pelvic Health PT Provider Locator'.

Pro Tip: Men can do Kegels too. Men can have pelvic health issues too. Several PTs who work in this specialty can help them too. This info might be useful for a loved one now, or later.

Pelvic pain is not normal. Ignoring it now can have lasting effects. If you still have pelvic pain or issues with incontinence at your six- to eight-week post-delivery OB checkup, you should schedule a visit with a pelvic floor therapist to address this.

You can actually schedule a post-partum PT evaluation, even in the absence of problems. All moms can ask for a check to prevent injuries, following the birth of a child. This will help you know that you're ready to return to exercise or sports.

The "fourth trimester" is a term referring to the postpartum period of time immediately following your delivery. It's not a catchy term, but a real thing that deserves the increase in attention it's gaining. Each postpartum mom has a different combination of emotional, physical and financial needs.

Maybe you needed help after #1 and didn't know to look, or where to look for some help. This is your reminder to ask for help when you need it.

Sometimes Baby #2 brings on issues, even when Baby #1 did not. Why? Think about all the extra daily tasks you're doing to take care of your first child(ren). Bending, lifting, cooking for them! Now your body is strained plus overworked. That's why.

MENTAL HEALTH

Have you ever laid awake in bed, wondering what your baby would look like? If breastfeeding is going to be hard? If your other relationships would lose their sparkle in comparison to the perfect human being you created? Are you already thinking ahead to when they're teenagers and you're going to have to be the strictest parent on the block because, "My House, My Rules?"

It's normal to feel overwhelmed with all the changes in your life. All the decisions you have to make. You wish you were a turtle and could draw your head into your thick, protective shell, or just hide under your blankets and wish the feelings away. From time to time, this comes with the territory.

If worries are dominating your life, please contact a professional for help. Counselors specialize in coaching you through any pre- or postpartum stress and depression. If talking it out isn't enough, they can prescribe lifesaving medicine or check the dose on something you're used to taking in case an update is what you need.

You are not an island. You are not alone. You are loved. There is help for you.

SOCIAL NETWORK

Find a group

If you don't know a lot of people in your area, or if you want to make friends with other new moms, find a group. Many hospitals have groups you can join with others having babies around the same time as you. You don't have to be a first-timer!

I didn't find a group of moms until my kids were pre-school age, and boy did I miss out! My other friends and neighbors have really tight bonds with friends they met in mom groups. So tight, that some remain group members even after their kids outgrow the pre-school years.

Some groups meet routinely at playgrounds or take turns at each other's houses. Some even exercise together. If you love to run, many cities and suburbs have groups that meet and run with their jogging strollers.

Did you ever do a Last Man Sprint (previously known as Indian Run) in gym class, or for an after-school sport? If you're super into fitness, you should try this with a stroller. Again, I missed the boat on this, but it was amazing to watch every week, looking out the window at the trail near work.

I did sign up for a local group, but the meeting times never worked out, so I never went. If you weren't able to find your community this way, consider the online options below.

If groups aren't really your thing, phone a friend. Or your mom. The phone works both ways. If you're thinking of someone you miss, or with whom you want to share your latest baby news, call them *today*.

Social Media Pages or Websites

Is time or distance holding you back from a face-to-face group? Find a group or message board online. You can bring up problems and get a consensus on solutions. Sometimes I just need back-up from someone who has "been there, done that" or is going through the same situation.

Just saying things out loud or asking in a small, judgment-free group helps you work through the ideas in your head.

I love working with and talking to people that have more experience than me. When talking out loud with someone, you can work out your own answer. In my case, they'd often laugh, because a lot of times I had my own answer the whole time. I just needed to say it out loud or have someone I like, and trust agree. I always wrap up those conversations with, "I'm glad we had this talk!"

If you've made it this far in the book, you already have a lot in common with the other readers who did the same. This is your official invitation to my private Facebook Moms group. www.pregnancypainbook.com/facebookfriends

Jump right in and get involved with the buddy system, or maybe just use it as a brain-break to post a funny/not-so-funny meme about the joys and pitfalls of pregnancy and being a mom. There's also a link in the back of the book.

But First, Pray
Many churches, synagogues, and temples have resources to help expectant or new mothers. Help can be financial, from a food pantry, counseling, or they may sponsor groups that meet routinely for an hour or two per week for a "semester."

These small groups can be the best—like free therapy! Larger communities and houses of worship may have more choices and opportunities. In many cases, you don't even have to be a member of the faith community to join. Do you have a friend that loves to share the joyful word? Ask them about group meetings and if they know of any moms that get together.

Excuses kept all my Pro Tips in my head for years! Because of getting into my first church group, I finally realized I was the girl to bring together these tips and share with all you mamas out there. They are to thank for this book, so just imagine what a few friends could do for you.

"If you wait until all the lights are 'green' before you leave home, you'll never get started on your trip...." ~Zig Ziglar

WEIGHT MANAGEMENT

Racing to the finish line for your target pregnancy weight? And it's not due to a swelling condition causing you to hold too much fluid?

Licensed nutritionists are your first point of help for this. Some large grocery stores have nutritionists that have weekly hours for a free consultation—or, alternately, you pay a fee for their time and get that same dollar amount back in store credit. It works out to be a free resource.

There are a million different diet lanes you can drive in. It could be Paleo, Whole30, vegan, on and on. I've used apps to count calories; I've taken the FedUp Challenge several times (no added sugar for ten days, a great reset button that is actually doable and safe while pregnant); and I've heeded the advice from a book called *How Not to Die.*[43]

Some days I'm vegan, some days I'm vegetarian, some days I'm not. Now I'm trending toward Dairy Free. I've done aspects of an internet challenge called 75 Hard. Do your research, and choose the one that best suits your lifestyle and needs. Each lane has its benefits.

Consider your and your family's schedule, tastes, values, and time. Make sure your diet provides you with the right amount of food or calories to support your body and your growing baby. The most important thing is to find something that is sustainable for you *and* your family. I've never stuck with an eating lifestyle that I did alone.

Chapter 13 Key Points
- o   Slow down on the stairs.
- o   Pelvic pain isn't normal. Call a therapist if incontinence or pain is ruining your day.
- o   If worries are dominating your life, call a counselor.
- o   Check out my Facebook Moms group, because it takes a village to raise a child.
- o   Choose a healthy eating lane, and find a friend to ride with you.
- o   Do ten Kegels right now.

CHAPTER FOURTEEN

NOT YOUR FIRST RODEO

Is there any difference between your first and second pregnancies? Or numbers three, four, five, etcetera? Anything new to know about your first weeks with baby *dos, tres, cuatro*, or *cinco*? In a word, *si*.

TIMELINE CHANGES

Back pain. Many times, pregnancy #1 is great! No pain. However, due to the relaxin stretching out your ligaments from before, the system is already weakened for the next baby. This might be your first time for back pain, or the gestational week that it starts could move waaaaaaay up, say, from week 28 to week 20.

In addition to your system being pre-weakened, what else is different? Oh yeah, you are bending down, lifting, and caring for your other child(ren). No strain there!

One fun thing about timelines is looking forward to when you'll jump into those fabulous, stretchy pregnancy pants again. My brain and body were ready several weeks sooner with my second pregnancy.

Those Are Kicks!

The bright side is, many times you feel your baby moving and kicking at an earlier week in successive pregnancies. Typically, you know what it feels like, or what to look for, which is awesome.

What I miss the most about carrying babies is when they kick or move. I always felt like there was an alien in my body taking control of major body functions. It also reminded me that I always had a buddy with me.

Bonus: If you talk to yourself like I do (role-playing two person conversations, narrating what I'm doing, or just general mutterings), when you get busted for talking to yourself, you can just say you're talking to your baby.

Attend all your prenatal appointments. Even though you've been through all your milestones before, and even if your previous pregnancy or pregnancies were uncomplicated, you need to check on the well-being of this baby. And of course, have all the ultrasounds recommended so you can sneak a peek at your beautiful, sweet babe.

THAT'S A BIG BABY

According to a study of 792 moms that delivered twice from 2005 to 2008, the second-born infants were on average 89 grams (.196 pounds AKA 3.14 ounces) heavier than the birthweight of their first born.[44]

That's not such good news if you pushed number one out with difficulty. My second was seven ounces bigger than my first. They have the same father, and they were both girls. Each baby arrived one day before their predicted due date, so time in-belly was the same.

Don't make the same bad food choices I did with #2. Eat smart. Hopefully doing so will help ensure that 3 ounces or 7 ounces doesn't tip the scale too, too much!

THE GEAR

A two-seat stroller is awesome if you actually need to leave the house and get anything done—that is, at a place that doesn't have shopping carts. Purse hooks for your stroller are also a must have, to keep important items close.

Ergo carrier. If you didn't really use one with the first kiddo, it's time to get it out of the box. Your older, energetic other kids need to run and play and learn outside, but your new baby isn't going to be running with them for a while. Learn to love your carrier.

HOW TO HOLD TWO

Now that your carrier is out of the box, let's talk about one person carrying two babies. You can make small moves without any gear holding two, but you're not going to get much done. And you may hurt yourself.

Serious stuff here: it's time to dial-in your baby-holding game.

Baby wearing is carrying your baby with a carrier, wrap, or device that leaves your hands and arms free. There's a big world out there on baby wearing. There's a ton of new options in recent years. A soft structured carrier (Ergo style), ring sling, Meh Dai, or a woven wrap all fit the wearer and baby a bit differently.

Ergo is still my go-to carrier, but like all things they fit everyone differently based on body type, age/size of baby, and even preferences the baby may have on how to be carried. Yes, it sounds crazy, but some

145

babies only like specific carriers. Each carrier is different and amazing in its own way.

I would call my friend Jami, an expert at babywearing. She has five kids aged seven years and under. She wears some babies! She's involved in a local baby-wearing club and gave me the scoop.

Many local clubs offer free meetings to try on carriers from their extensive library. Baby wearing might seem straightforward, but very often caregivers visit and complain about the carriers being uncomfortable. A club of moms with recent experience can make some helpful tweaks, which can make all the difference.

For a small annual membership fee, some clubs allow you to borrow one or two carriers every month and not worry about spending so much money on one carrier that you might not love during your baby wearing journey.

Ideally, everyone would go to a meeting and get hands-on help finding what works best for them. The baby-wearing community is all over the United States, and it is reasonably easy to find a local meeting. And, bonus: now you found a new club of moms you can add to your new circle of friends going through this chapter of life with you.

OK, so back to two at once. There are specific carriers to use with twins, or you can pair carriers together. You can put your toddler on your back and your baby on your front to balance your center of gravity as best as you can. Use this trick with shopping, or while caring for that infant.

Remember those sit-to-stand exercises? Now that you have pounds and pounds of babies strapped to your body, those rock-solid legs are ready to help you carry!

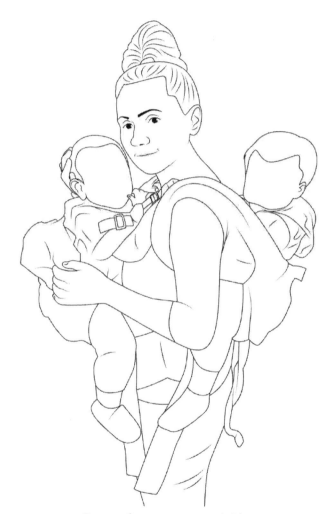

Posture for carrying two children

TO SPRINKLE, OR NOT TO SPRINKLE

Did someone offer to host a sprinkle in your and your baby's honor? A sprinkle is a mini version of a shower. People figure you have the expensive gear, and that you've had a big party for another baby, so plans and expectations are typically more relaxed for baby #2.

I am a planner! We knew we were having a girl with both pregnancies, thanks to the anatomy scan. We had two girls in under two years. I'm not one for the spotlight, so I said "no, thank you" to a sprinkle from our family.

Just say "yes".

You will always need diapers and gift cards to restock your favorite baby must-haves. Having a baby is a big deal. Not just for the work your body is doing, but for the love and joy it's going to bring to everyone that's ready to love your baby.

During my last week of work before Baby #2 arrived, a low-key, surprise brunch sprinkle was planned. It was cancelled due to bad weather (January in Maryland, go figure). I realized then how disappointed I was that I missed out!

Just say "yes" to a sprinkle!

Chapter 14 Key Points
- o   Check out your local baby wearing club for a loaner.
- o   Just say "yes" to a sprinkle.
- o   Do ten Kegels right now.

You Got This

Quit Trying to Be Perfect

Thank you for reading. I hope you learned something by picking up this book. I hope you look at baby gear and your posture differently and move with more understanding of how to take care of you and your body, so you can focus on all the joy happening in your life right now.

I have so many "funny/not-so-funny" memories that writing has conjured, like the first diaper we changed resulted in tar-like baby poo on the brand-new, turquoise curtains. Holy Poop! It took a long time to get those curtains in the wash. In a moment, the perfect nest I posted on Facebook weeks before was, "lived in," poo and all.

Raising a baby is a messy, beautiful journey, so enjoy it. Try to make time to live in the moment. Take a look around.

Major milestones in my life really opened my eyes to a new level of judgement, drama, grudges, and feelings that get hurt. Marriage, making choices for your baby, making choices for your growing child, all of it. With pregnancy and raising a child, there are literally thousands of choices to make. With some, you have to think fast. Others you worry over for quite a while.

Life brings you surprises every day. This pregnancy itself might have been a surprise, but here you are. You're making choices for you and your baby. Lots of choices.

Some choices will feel like epic fails. Just remember, when you don't win, you learn!

Quit judging. We compare ourselves to others too often.[45] Which is better? A stay-at-home-mom, part-time mom, full-time working mom? Each scenario comes with its own pros and cons. Some moms have a choice from those options; some moms don't.

Regardless of your circumstances, if you made the decision to read this book, I know you're a mom who is eager to do what is best for her baby.

It's not unusual to feel burdened or crushed by society's expectations to be the "best" mom. Quit comparing yourself to moms that seem like they have it all figured out. Quit trying to be perfect at sleep schedules, making homemade food, or hitting prenatal yoga poses.

Think of all the things you do to take care of you, your partner, your future babysitters, and your baby. You're setting your baby up for the love it needs.

This baby is the baby you were meant to love. Whether you're the birth (AKA biological) mom, adopted mom, dad, grandma, grandpa, or excitedly expectant Auntie or Godparent of a new baby, you were chosen to be in this baby's life.

Be intentional. This baby needs love and support. Love those in your life that are part of this journey. Love yourself. Love your baby.

You are the one for the job. And you can do it.

BONUS

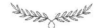

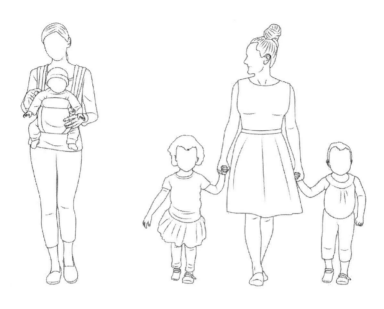

So, what's next? After our physical therapy clients graduate with us, it's never, "I hope I never see you again." I tell them, "Let me know if anything comes up for you later." The best way to reach my readers near and far is online. To that end, I have created www.pregnancypainbook.com. It's a site full of practical tips and links covered in this book.

Looking for step-by-step instructions on the exercises I covered? www.pregnancypainbook.com/exercises gives you every little tip and reminder to help you do the exercises correctly at home. Dive deep to supplement the book or Cheat Sheet.

Need a quick list of the gear you need to share with someone or add to your registry?

I've put all these in one easy place to find:
www.pregnancypainbook.com/gear

I will continue to update this list as the latest and greatest gear comes to market even if items aren't mentioned here. It is a page you will want to visit to stay connected, so have a look.

Looking for that Facebook group from Chapter 13? The official group name and link is here www.pregnancypainbook.com/facebookfriends

Hope to see you there soon!

ACKNOWLEDGEMENTS

There are numerous people who believed in me and helped me put all these words on paper. This book would not have been possible without the positivity, accountability, wisdom, and creativity of the following people.

Chandler Bolt, Chad Aleo, Ellaine Ursuy, Lise Cartwright, Marcy Pusey, Sean Sumner, PT and the entire Self Publishing School community.

Content Contributors: Amanda Fleming, MPT, Jami Funk-Wilbanks, Jessica Wright, Maureen Webb, DPT & Meghan Swenck, DPT, WCS.

Disclaimer: Hugh Farrell, Esq & Laura Thomas, Esq at Davis Agnor Rapaport & Skalny.

Draft Readers: Christina Ewald, Jennifer Turner, Lisa Evans, Randi LaBorde, Sarah Linden-Brooks, and T.J. Sanner.

Content & Copy Editing: Qat Wanders and her team at Wandering Words Media.

Proofreading: Dr. Sherri L. Foster.

Cover Design: Ceb Atölye Graphics featuring floral vector art from Freepik.

Illustrations: Budiawan.

Formatting: Rachael Cox.

Chad Madden, Carl Mattiola, all the members, staff & partners of Breakthrough Physical Therapy Marketing.

My entire fam at Atlas Physical Therapy, Glen Burnie, Maryland.

C.J. Canby, Dana Stafford, Jenn Farrelly, Leanna Canby, all the staff, volunteers, and friends with Lighthouse Church, Glen Burnie, Maryland.

I cannot thank them enough for the impact they've had on my life.

ABOUT THE AUTHOR

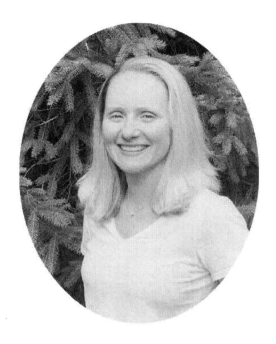

Laura Sanner is living her dream of helping people. The senior message she wrote in her high school yearbook was to "become a physical therapist and live a happy life." She wrote this book to help her readers experience more of the day-to-day joy and happiness that being pregnant should bring.

Laura loves music, Halloween, cooking, sports, and spending time with family and friends. By day you can find her working hands-on in her Physical Therapy clinic in Maryland, and by night, making memories with her husband T.J. and their two daughters.

REFERENCES

I try to share what works. My methods are rooted in scientific research published in professional journals. In your search to fact-check ideas from this book, look for legitimate peer-reviewed journal articles. I've also gleaned some solid life-lessons from authored books. My book was compiled using information and ideas from the following sources:

[1] Warland J et al. Modifying Maternal Sleep Position in Late Pregnancy Through Positional Therapy: A Feasibility Study. *J Clin Sleep Med.* 2018;14(8):1387-1397.

[2] Exactly How Bad Is It to Sleep on Your Back When You're Pregnant? https://health.clevelandclinic.org/exactly-how-bad-is-it-to-sleep-on-your-back-when-youre-pregnant/. Accessed June 2020.

[3] Nelson, P: Pulmonary gas embolism in pregnancy and the puerperium. *Obstet Gynecol Surv* 15, 1960.

[4] Bassett DR, et al. Pedometer-measured physical activity and health behaviors in U.S. adults. *Med Sci Sports Exerc.* 42(10):1819-25, 2010.

[5] Cook SD, et al. Shock absorption characteristics of running shoes. *Am J Sports Med.* 13(4):248-253, 1985.

[6] Klinich KD, et al. Fetal outcome in motor-vehicle crashes: effects of crash characteristics and maternal restraint. *Am J Obstet Gynecol* 2008; 198:450.

[7] Katonis et al. Pregnancy-related low back pain. *Hippokratia.* 2011 Jul-Sep; 15(3): 205–210.

[8] Khosrawi, S and Maghrouri, R. The prevalence and severity of carpal tunnel syndrome during pregnancy. *Adv Biomed Res.* 2012; 1: 43.

[9] Boissonnault JS and Blaschak. Incidence of diastasis recti abdominis during the childbearing year. *Physical Therapy.* 1988;68: 1082-1086.

[10] Gluppe SL, et al. Effect of a Postpartum Training Program on the Prevalence of Diastasis Recti Abdominis in Postpartum Primiparous Women: A Randomized Controlled Trial. *Phys Ther.* 2018;98(4):260–268.

[11] Mohamed A, et al. Effect of Kinesio Taping on Diastasis Recti. *Med. J. Cairo Univ.,* Vol. 85, No. 6, September: 2289-2296, 2017.

[12] Thélin CS, Richter JE. Review article: The management of heartburn during pregnancy and lactation. *Aliment Pharmacol Ther.* 2020;51(4):421-434.

[13] ACOG committee opinion. Exercise during pregnancy and the postpartum period. Number 267, January 2002. American College of Obstetricians and Gynecologists. *Int J Gynaecol Obstet.* 2002 Apr;77(1):79-81.

[14] Exercise in Pregnancy and the Postpartum Period. Joint guidelines, Society of Obstetricians and Gynacologists of Canada and the Canadian Society for Exercise Physiology. *J Obstet Gynaecol Can* 25(6):516-522, 2003.

[15] Clapp, JF. Exercise and fetal health. *J Dev Physiol* 15:9, 1991.

[16] Koshino T. Management of regular exercise in pregnant women. *J Nippon Med Sch.* 2003 Apr;70(2):124-8.

[17] Mottola MF. Components of Exercise Prescription and Pregnancy. *Clin Obstet Gynecol.* 2016; 59(3): 552-558.

[18] Clapp JF. Long-term outcome after exercising throughout pregnancy: fitness and cardiovascular risk. *Am J Obstet Gynecol.* 199(5): 489, 2008.

[19] Ostgaard, HC, et al: Reduction of back and posterior pelvic pain in pregnancy. *Spine* 19:894, 1994.

[20] Clapp, JF. Exercise during pregnancy: a clinical update. *Clin Sports Med* 19(2): 273, 2000.

[21] Lewis, Paul B. et al. Muscle Soreness and Delayed-Onset Muscle Soreness. *Clinics in Sports Medicine*, Volume 31, Issue 2, 255 – 262.

[22] Exercise in Pregnancy and the Postpartum Period. Joint guidelines, Society of Obstetricians and Gynacologists of Canada and the Canadian Society for Exercise Physiology. *J Obstet Gynaecol Can* 25(6):516-522, 2003.

[23] Lorenzetti, Silvio et al. "How to squat? Effects of various stance widths, foot placement angles and level of experience on knee, hip and trunk motion and loading." *BMC sports science, medicine & rehabilitation* vol. 10 14. 17 Jul. 2018.

[24] Waters, Thomas R et al. Provisional recommended weight limits for manual lifting during pregnancy. *Human factors* vol. 56,1 (2014): 203-14.

[25] D'Lima DD, et al. Knee joint forces: prediction, measurement, and significance. *Proceedings of the Institution of Mechanical Engineers. Part H, Journal of engineering in medicine* vol. 226,2 (2012): 95-102.

[26] Franklin, Ashley et al. Rowers' Self-Reported Behaviors, Attitudes, and Safety Concerns Related to Exercise, Training, and Competition During Pregnancy. *Cureus* vol. 9,8 e1534. 1 Aug. 2017.

[27] Özgüven HN, Berme N. An experimental and analytical study of impact forces during human jumping. *Journal of Biomechanics*. Vol. 21,12 (1988): 1061-1066.

[28] Tenforde AS et al. Running habits of competitive runners during pregnancy and breastfeeding. *Sports Health*. 2015 Mar;7(2):172-6.

[29] Kisner C et al. Therapeutic Exercise: Foundations and Techniques. Chapter: Special Areas of Therapeutic Exercise: Women's Health: Obstetrics and Pelvic Floor. 7th edition. Oct 2017.

[30] Mørkved, S, et al: Pelvic floor muscle training during pregnancy to prevent urinary incontinence: a single-blind randomized controlled trial. *Obstet Gynecol* 101(2):313-319, 2003.

[31] Brearley AL, et al. Pregnant Women Maintain Body Temperatures Within Safe Limits During Moderate-Intensity Aqua-Aerobic Classes Conducted in Pools Heated up to 33 Degrees Celsius: An Observational Study. *J Physiother.* 2015 Oct;61(4):199-203.

[32] Nieuwenhuijsen MJ. Distribution and determinants of trihalomethane concentrations in indoor swimming pools. *Occup Environ Med.* 2002 Apr;59(4):243-7.

[33] Field, T. Pregnant Women Benefit From Massage Therapy. *J Psychosom Obstet Gynaecol.* Mar 1999;20(1):31-8.

[34] Nelson, P: Pulmonary gas embolism in pregnancy and the puerperium. *Obstet Gynecol Surv* 15, 1960.

[35] Fainting. American College of Emergency Physicians. http://www.emergencycareforyou.org/EmergencyManual/WhatToDoInMedicalEmergency/Default.aspx?id=240. Accessed Apr 2020.

[36] Bae S, et al. The effects of kinesio taping on potential in chronic low back pain patients anticipatory postural control and cerebral cortex. *J Phys Ther Sci.* 2013;25(11):1367-1371.

[37] Karp, Harvey. The Happiest Baby on the Block: The New Way to Calm Crying and Help Your Newborn Baby Sleep Longer. Oct 2015.

[38] A Guide to Handling Patients, Fourth Edition. Published by: IMPACC.

[39] Cluver C, et al. Interventions for Helping to Turn Term Breech Babies to Head First Presentation When Using External Cephalic Version. *Cochrane Database Syst Rev.* 2015 Feb 9.

[40] Kaufman T. Evolution of the birth plan. *J Perinat Educ.* 2007;16(3):47–52.

[41] Ranjbaran et al. Effect of Massage Therapy on Labor Pain Reduction in Primiparous Women: A Systematic Review and Meta-analysis of Randomized Controlled Clinical Trials in Iran. *Iran J Nurs Midwifery Res.* 2017 Jul-Aug; 22(4): 257–261.

[42] Messelink, Bert et al. Standardization of terminology of pelvic floor muscle function and dysfunction: report from the pelvic floor clinical assessment group of the International Continence Society. *Neurourology and urodynamics*, vol. 24,4: 374-80, 2005.

[43] Greger, M and Stone, G. How Not To Die: Discover the Foods Scientifically Proven to Prevent and Reverse Disease. Apr 2016.

[44] Bacci, S et al. Differences in Birthweight Outcomes: A Longitudinal Study Based on Siblings. *Int J Environ Res Public Health.* 2014 Jun; 11(6): 6472–6484.

[45] Connolly, Jessica. You Are the Girl for the Job: Daring to Believe the God Who Calls You. Sep 2019.

URGENT PLEA!

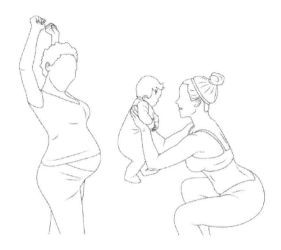

Thank You for Reading My Book!

I love hearing what you have to say,
and I really appreciate all your feedback.

I need your input to make future editions of this book better.

Let me know which Tips you found most helpful or if any of this
information stirred up questions I didn't answer.

Please leave me a helpful review letting me know what you thought of
my book.

Thank you very much!

~Dr. Laura